RAPID W  S
HYl

Emotional Eating And Deep Sleep Meditation
For Men And Women To Change Habits And
Lose Weight Fast. Improve Your Self-Esteem
With Motivational Affirmations

Jessica Williams

Table of Contents

BOOK 1 :

RAPID WEIGHT LOSS HYPNOSIS AND DEEP SLEEP MEDITATION

SELF-HYPNOSIS FOR MEN AND WOMEN TO CHANGE EATING HABITS AND LOSE WEIGHT WITH GUIDED MEDITATION AND MOTIVATIONAL AFFIRMATIONS

Introduction

Need to lose 5 pounds in a week? The right combination of hypnosis and deep sleep meditation can help you burn more calories while you sleep. We'll also teach you how to get into the deepest stage of slumber easily so that you wake up feeling refreshed without ever experiencing the negative effects of being deprived of oxygen. Ready to learn more? Follow this link.

Hypnosis is among the most popular weight loss techniques, as 50% or more of dieters who use it are successful at achieving their goals. That's why hypnosis is so appealing to many people, and it's becoming more popular. I've been a hypnotist for over 20 years, and many of my clients are also hypnotists.

Because the use of deep sleep hypnosis is fairly new, there isn't much research about it yet. I'm hoping this book will bring you new ideas about ways to use hypnosis to quickly lose weight while you sleep. If you're already using deep sleep hypnosis in your practice, that's wonderful! Please share any new experiences or successes that you have had with it in our forum.

Deep Sleep Hypnosis

Deep sleep hypnosis, as the name implies, uses hypnotic suggestions to get you into a deep slumber. Your body becomes less aware of its physical limitations, which allows you to lose weight without experiencing the negative effects of starvation like it does with traditional dieting. It's also very good for weight loss. And if you're already following a diet and exercising in your daily routine, then deep sleep hypnosis is perfect for just the transition from dieting to weight maintenance.

As you lose weight, your metabolism slows down. This causes the body to use less energy, and your body has to eat less and use stored fat to generate the energy it needs. It's a vicious cycle that almost all dieters soon find themselves in. But with deep sleep hypnosis, you don't hunger for food because your metabolism has slowed down enough so that you can still burn stored fat for energy.

The trick is getting into a deep enough state of slumber so that oxygen deprivation doesn't wake you up before the hypnosis can take effect. That's where I was able to learn about this new way of using hypnosis for weight loss. I have worked with many people who have tried deep sleep hypnosis and had great results, but they could never get "into" it because they were too conscious. That's why I created the "deep sleep induction script." It helps the body to go into deep slumber more quickly so that you wake up feeling refreshed without having to suffer from the negative effects of deprivation of oxygen.

There are two parts to this article. First, I'll show you how hypnosis works for weight loss, and then I'll teach you how to use a hypnotic induction script that makes it easier for your unconscious mind to get into a deep sleep.

How hypnosis helps you lose weight

The key to weight loss hypnosis is that your conscious mind isn't aware that it's happening, so your body can burn fatter than it otherwise would. I'm sure you've had the experience of lying down and feeling sleepy, and then suddenly remembering that you need to get up to do something. And then you're wide awake again. That's your conscious mind catching onto what's happening, it doesn't want to fall asleep, so it tells the body to wake up. And this happens over and over until you finally do fall asleep.

That's why you need to make sure that your unconscious mind can get into a deep sleep quickly. Once it does, your body will burn stored fat for energy, and the weight loss will happen naturally. When you wake up, you'll feel refreshed without any of the negative consequences of deprivation of oxygen or food.

Using a hypnotic induction script to get into deep sleep hypnosis

Here's how a typical session goes using deep sleep hypnosis: First, I give the client suggestions about becoming more relaxed as he or she listens to my voice. Then I've got the client to listen to a recording that uses binaural beats to help with relaxation and slow the brain waves down into a pattern associated with deep slumber. I've them listen to the recording twice, and then we take a break for 5 to 10 minutes.

While waiting for the client to return, I keep up with the suggestions of feeling more relaxed. I use a program on my computer that plays white noise so that the client will have no awareness of my voice as he or she falls asleep. This is critical to success because if you can see me or hear me, you will become conscious of your surroundings and wake up.

When the client returns, I begin giving suggestions about deep sleep hypnosis as he or she listens to another recording of binaural beats while lying down in bed. This triple induction has been very effective for helping people to get very deeply into hypnosis, even those who never thought they could before.

Writing the induction script

The deep sleep induction script is extremely effective and will work for anyone. It's very easy to write this yourself. Just follow the steps below, and you'll be on your way!

First, decide what you want your client to focus on while in deep sleep hypnosis. It could be weight loss, a better relationship with a spouse or significant other, or just getting more restful sleep. Whatever it is that you want them to focus on during hypnosis, write it down. Then you need to come up with three suggestions that the client will believe when they are in deep sleep hypnosis. These are suggestions about deep sleep.

Once you've got your idea of what you want your client to focus on during hypnosis, go to a website like binauralbeats.com and listen to some music at different brain wave frequencies. This site has recordings that use binaural beats while playing white noise, this is how I help my clients get into a deep slumber for weight loss hypnosis. It's very effective. Once you've found a frequency of binaural beats that sounds good, use that as the background for your recording.

Create a voice recording on your computer with your script and have it playing while you play the binaural beats in the background. You can set up multiple recordings if you want to be able to play them back at the same time, but it makes sense to do this only if you will be using it frequently or if you're going to train someone else to do this for you.

When you are about to help the client into a deep sleep, simply say the binaural beat parts in your recording while continuing to talk about the things that you want him or her to focus on during the deep sleep. For weight loss hypnosis, I usually ask them to think about getting slim and trim. When they are in a state of deep slumber, they will focus on this thought of wanting to be slim and trim while they fall asleep.

Once you've gotten them into a relaxed state where they believe your suggestions, tell them to get ready for that dreamlike state of deep, restful sleep that many people dream about when they are going to lay down for a vacation or just need some rest. You can do this by telling them to remain relaxed and not to try to control their thoughts. Tell them that they will be in a dreamlike state that while they're listening and falling asleep.

This takes practice. So, if you make your first recording use it as an opportunity to see how well it works and if you're getting the results you want for yourself or your clients. Practice once or twice daily so that you don't find yourself standing in front of a client without being able to do anything at all for them. You should be able to hear the difference, even after only one time of getting this right, especially if you're trying to help someone with weight loss hypnosis.

If you suspect that you have never achieved the results you desire, or if your clients have stopped responding to hypnosis with weight loss and are in other ways not responding to your suggestions, then you might need to listen to this recording again as well.

Chapter 1 - Hypnosis Explained

The Origin of Hypnosis

There are numerous inconsistencies throughout the entire existence of hypnosis. Its set of experiences is somewhat similar to attempting to discover the historical backdrop of relaxing. Hypnosis is a general quality that was worked upon entering the world. It has been capable and shared by each human since forever ago. It has quite recently been in the previous few decades that we are starting to get this. Hypnosis hasn't changed in 1,000,000 years. How we get it and how we control it has changed a great deal.

Hypnosis has consistently been encircled by misinterpretations and fantasies. Regardless of being utilized clinically and all the exploration that has been done, some keep on being frightened by the suspicion that hypnosis is otherworldly. Numerous individuals feel that hypnosis is an advanced development that spread through networks that trusted in the otherworldly during the 70s and 80s. Since the mid-1800s, hypnosis was utilized in the United States. It has progressed with the assistance of clinicians like Alfred Binet, Pierre Janet, and Sigmund Freud, and others. Hypnosis can be found in old occasions and has been examined by current analysts, doctors, and therapists.

Hypnosis's starting points can't be isolated from brain science and western medication. Most antiquated societies from Roman, Greek, Egyptian, Indian, Chinese, Persian, and Sumerian utilized hypnosis. In Greece and Egypt, individuals who were wiped out would go to the spots that recuperated. These were known as dream sanctuaries or rest sanctuaries where individuals could be restored with hypnosis.

The Sanskrit book called "The Law of Manu" portrayed degrees of hypnosis, for example, rest strolling, dream rest, and delight rest in old India.

The most punctual proof of hypnosis was found in the Egyptian Ebers Papyrus that dated back to 1550 B.C. Minister/doctors rehashed ideas while treating patients. They would have a patient look at metal circles and enter a daze. This is presently called eye obsession.

During the Middle Ages, sovereigns and rulers figured they could mend with the Royal Touch. These healings can be ascribed to divine forces. Before individuals started to get hypnosis, the terms hypnotism or attraction would be utilized to depict this kind of recuperating.

Paracelsus, the Swiss doctor, started utilizing magnets to recuperate. He didn't utilize a sacred relic or heavenly touch. This kind of recuperating was all the while being utilized during the 1700s. A Jesuit minister, Maximillian Hell, was acclaimed for recuperating utilizing attractive steel plates. Franz Mesmer, an Austrian doctor, found he could send individuals into a daze without the utilization of magnets. He sorted out the recuperating power that came from inside himself or an imperceptible liquid that occupied the room. He felt that "creature attraction" could be moved from the patient to healer by a strange etheric liquid. This hypothesis is so off-base. It depended on thoughts that were current during the time, explicitly Isaac Newton's hypothesis of gravity.

Mesmer built up a strategy for hypnosis that was given to his devotees. Mesmer would perform enlistments by connecting his patients together by a rope that the creature attraction could ignore. He would likewise wear a

18

shroud and play music on a glass harmonica while this was going on. The picture that a subliminal specialist was a supernatural figure returns to this.

These practices prompted his defeat, and for time trancelike influence was considered risky for anybody to have as a vocation. The reality is that hypnosis works. The nineteenth century was brimming with individuals who were hoping to comprehend and apply it.

Marquis de Puysegur, an understudy of Mesmer, was an effective magnetist who initially utilized hypnosis called insomnia or sleepwalking. Puysegur's adherents called themselves experimentalists. Their work perceived that fixes didn't come from magnets, however, an imperceptible source.

Abbe Faria, an Indo-Portuguese cleric, did hypnosis research in India during 1813. He went to Paris and contemplated hypnosis with Puysegur. He felt that hypnosis or attraction wasn't what recuperated, however, the force that was created from inside the psyche.

His methodology was what aided open the psychotherapy hypnosis-focused school called Nancy School. The Nancy School said that hypnosis was a wonder welcomed on by the force of idea and not from the attraction.

This school was established by a French nation specialist, Ambroise-Auguste Liebeault. He was known as the dad of current hypnotherapy. He thought hypnosis was mental and had nothing to do with attraction. He examined the comparative characteristics of daze and rest and saw that hypnosis was an expression that could be welcomed on my idea.

His book Sleep and Its Analogous States was imprinted in 1866. The accounts and compositions about his fixes pulled in Hippolyte Bernheim to visit him.

Bernheim was a renowned nervous system specialist who was suspicious of Liebeault, yet once he noticed Liebault, he was interested to the point that he surrendered interior medication and turned into a hypnotic specialist. Bernheim carried Liebeault's plans to the clinical world with Suggestive Therapeutics that showed hypnosis as a science. Bernheim and Liebeault were the trailblazers of psychotherapy. Indeed, even today, hypnosis is as yet seen as a wonder.

The pioneers of brain research considered hypnosis in Paris and Nancy Schools. Pierre Janey created speculations of horrible memory, separation, and oblivious cycles considered hypnosis with Bernheim in Charcot in Paris and Nancy. Sigmund Freud considered hypnosis with Charcot and noticed both Liebeault and Bernheim. Freud began rehearsing hypnosis in 1887. Hypnosis was basic in his created therapy.

During the time that hypnosis was being designed, a few doctors started utilizing hypnosis for sedation. Recamier, in 1821 worked while utilizing hypnosis as sedation. John Elliotson, a British specialist in 1834, presented the stethoscope in England. He revealed doing a few effortless activities by utilizing hypnosis. A Scottish specialist, James Esdaile, did more than 345 significant and 2,000 minor tasks by utilizing hypnosis during the 1840s and 1850s. James Braid, a Scottish ophthalmologist, concocted current hypnotism.

Twist originally utilized the term apprehensive rest or neuro-trance induction that became hypnosis or trancelike influence. Mesh went to a show of La Fontaine, the French attraction in 1841. He scorned the Mesmerists' thoughts and proposed that hypnosis was mental. He was quick to rehearse psychosomatic medication. He attempted to say that hypnosis was simply zeroing in on one thought.

Hypnosis was progressed by the Nancy School and is as yet a term we use today. The focal point of hypnosis moved out of Europe and into America. Here it had numerous leap forwards in the twentieth century. Hypnosis was a famous wonder that since more accessible to typical individuals who were not specialists.

Hypnosis's style changed, as well. It was not, at this point, direct guidelines from a powerful figure; all things being equal; it turned out to be even more a tolerant and backhanded style of daze that depended on unpretentious language designs. This was achieved by Milton H. Erickson. Utilizing hypnosis for the speedy treatment of injury and wounds during WWI, WWII, and Korea prompted another interest in hypnosis in psychiatry and dentistry.

Hypnosis began getting more functional and was considered as a device for aiding mental trouble. Advances in mind imaging and neurological science, alongside Ivan Tyrrell and Joe Griffin's work, have helped resolve a few discussions. These British therapists connected hypnosis to Rapid Eye Movement and carried hypnosis into the domain of everyday encounters. The idea of typical awareness can be seen better as daze expresses that we continually go all through.

There are still individuals who believe that hypnosis is a kind of force held by the mysterious even today. Individuals that accept hypnosis can handle minds or perform supernatural occurrences are sharing the perspectives that have been around for many years. The set of experiences that have been recorded is rich with looks at practices and antiquated customs that resemble present-day hypnosis. The Hindu Vedas have recuperating passes. Antiquated Egypt has its otherworldly messages. These practices were utilized for strict functions, such as speaking with spirits and divine beings. We need to recall that what individuals see as the mystery was science at its best at that time. It was doing likewise as present-day science was doing now, attempting to fix human sicknesses by expanding our insight.

Discovering the historical backdrop of hypnosis resembles looking for something that is directly in our view. We can start to perceive the truth about it, a marvel that is a confounded piece of human life. Hypnosis's future is to totally understand our characteristic mesmerizing capacities and the potential we as a whole hold inside us.

Chapter 2 - Make Wiser Choices, Thrill Your Soul

Making you feel happier than you at any point have. You will feel surer, enabled, and stimulated.

Presently you are starting to feel increasingly relaxed... I will ask you to imagine a beautiful white light encompassing you from head to toe... Wrapping you in consoling warmth ... (Pause).

This is your safe space. Your own little air pocket. You can venture into this air pocket each time you feel focused or uncertain, when you are searching for answers, or essentially to rest and get back to yourself.

Presently on my check, this air pocket will start to float... 1, 2, 3 ... it lifts you up tenderly... (pause) 4, 5, 6... (pause) you love this floaty inclination.... 7,8, 9.... Carrying you increasingly elevated... (pause) 10 the air pocket arrives at a delicate stop... You discover you are on a boat at sea... It is evening, and candle flickers tossing shadows on the walls of the boat's cabin... You notice the beautiful sundown and the last rays of the setting sun and can't help yet feel a profound peace... (pause).

You walk towards the candle and notice a wooden chest... It is somewhat open, and you catch a brief look at something shimmering ... (pause) You draw nearer and open the chest... And to your amazement, it is loaded up with dazzling gems.

You stare in stand amazed at the staggering array of glimmering diamonds... You believe they could have superpowers and feel a shiver of energy stumble into your body. (Pause)

The principal thing that catches your eye is a gleaming Emerald… You get it and hold it in two hands… You feel it pulsating magically…. This Emerald represents your food choices … As you hold it, you realize that it gives you intelligence and control, the order you need to not surrender to temptation, and reach for solace food when you feel annoyed, drained, or low. (Pause) You currently realize that each time you feel this way, you will basically reach for this gem or the idea (pause)

And instead of picking unhealthy snack alternatives… Lousy nourishment. singed and sugar-filled stuff … You will pick healthier food varieties… You are presently acutely aware of the fact that lousy nourishment simply fills you with void calories that make you gain weight and make you feel heavy and lazy… When you pick healthy food, you feel more energy and stay at a healthy weight. (Pause) As you are focusing on this beautiful Emerald, you notice it begins to break up into your hands and integrate into you. You feel invigorated and happy… You feel your blood clean and course through your veins… Any squares caused by an unhealthy eating routine, and eating patterns start to disintegrate with the energy of this gem and your freshly discovered purpose. (Pause) Next, you get a sparkling Yellow Sapphire, you are awestruck by its beauty, getting it, you realize it radiates warmth, and you start to feel loaded up with conviction. (Pause) This gem reminds you to stay consistent with your best self…

You realize how frequently you have stood in your own specific manner by weakening your determination and reaching for unhealthy food to make yourself feel good. As that beautiful Sapphire starts to pulsate and break up into your palms, you realize that you will never have to repeat these past mistakes… (Pause) Here on, you will always have a clear image of your dream body to you, and you presently have the courage it takes to quietness cravings and fills your body with just healthy food sources at the correct occasions. You will never again allow transient cravings to hinder your drawn-out goals, wellness. and prosperity! (pause).

It has become extremely clear to you that the key to managing one's food intake is down to being focused and regulating our cravings. Now and then. we have had the opportunity to swear off certain cravings to achieve the body of our dreams. (Pause).

You have already made steps in your wellness venture on this boat at this very moment. (pause).

Presently you get another shocking, gleaming gem… this one is a Ruby…

Radiating light and inspiration, you feel an incredible energy and appreciate simply holding it for a couple of moments (pause).

It dawns on you that you, at this point, don't have to feel overpowered and defenseless…

You actually have total control over your psyche and the choices you make… you choose what you eat, when you eat, and most importantly, how you feel when you eat. (Pause) You watch as the Ruby breaks down into your palms and feel its beautiful cherishing energy course through your veins it is the energy absorbed into your body. (Pause).

Presently you reach for a sparkling clear diamond … almost blinding in its brilliance… as you hold it affectionately in your palms you feel its clarity and energy … (pause).

You are loaded up with an added realization that you should be in a calm frame of the brain when you eat, so your food can be all around processed, and you just eat as much as you need to. (Pause)

You hold the diamond for a brief period longer (pause), and now watching it break down into your palms, you feel its calm clarity radiate through your whole body...

Presently your whole body starts to drone and radiates with the light and energy of the gems, you appreciate the invigorating inclination it radiates in your body and the calm, clarity you experience. (Pause) Now you turn upward and notice the lights are on, in your cabin on the boat...

You are as yet sailing joyfully on a very calm ocean. You notice an ice chest in the corner. You walk ready and open the entryway; you see all your favorite lousy nourishments... on one rack... and healthy food choices on another....

You are loaded up with another purpose and determination ... (you can feel all the jewel's energy pulsating unequivocally through you.). (Pause) You take this low-quality nourishment and step out onto the deck... you lay the food out across the deck for the gulls to feast on... it will make a fine supper for them... you realize you have lost all your taste for lousy nourishment, you currently know the nutritional value and benefits you can get from a healthy eating regimen. (Pause) As you scatter the food across the deck, you start to feel engaged, and you realize you are also freeing yourself of your appetite for lousy nourishment. You take your time scattering the food across the wide deck. watching the seagulls jump and feast... and with each offer of your hand, you feel yourself relinquishing your cravings forever. (Pause)

You return inside the cabin, and you choose a healthy meal, green leafy vegetables, healthy proteins, and entire food varieties... you realize it tastes heavenly and tops you off rather rapidly. (Pause)

You are shocked and charmed by how stimulated and healthy you feel and make a guarantee to proceed to always eat healthily. You feel very grateful for this new awareness and resolve and appeal to your psyche brain to help you every day to make astute choices. You realize that with a little control and center it's easy to do. (Pause)

You see yourself at family gatherings and social occasions... casually picking healthy food and smaller segments. You see yourself glancing very hot in your new smaller estimated clothes. things you wouldn't dare to take a gander at in the past ... (Pause)

You feel the appreciative glances from people around you and realize this is a far better inclination than the solace you got from eating shoddy nourishment.

You simply realize that you will be making healthier choices here on. (Pause) As you appreciate this sensation of satisfaction, and prosperity ... the lazy swaying of the boat across the ocean waves... the setting sun, and the indigo skies...

You take a second to acknowledge your freshly discovered awareness, you thank your psyche mind for showing you so much, and you ask it to assist you with remembering what you learned today always. (Pause)

Hold that feeling ... in a second, we will bring you back into the current second... Feel that beautiful energy bubble envelope you from head to toe and on my check... (pause)

10, 9, 8... the air pocket lifts you far up into the clouds... (pause) 7,6,5 ... tenderly carrying you, increasingly elevated. lighter than ever... 4, 3, 2.... You begin to dive... and 1... Eyes open... wide awake at this point. Wriggle your fingers and toes, stretch if you need to you are back right now

Chapter 3 - Diets Alone Cannot Solve Weight Problem

Do you realize that diet alone cannot solve the weight problem? Here are a couple of things you ought to do to guarantee that you accomplish that weight you have consistently longed for:

Partaking in a significant and all-around arranged exercise will most likely add to your prosperity while in transit to accomplishing your objective of losing pointless weight in other to appreciate a better life. There are some valuable tips here that can assist you with utilizing the force of activity.

Think about Taking Part in Workouts

Taking part in a sensible measure of activity is perhaps the best approach to shed pounds. Standard exercise will assist you with keeping abundance fats from amassing in your body. This will prompt a slow and reliable deficiency of weight. Note: in any case, that short, ordinary exercise is more successful than delayed exercise at diminishing weight. You can think about beginning with little activities like energetic strolling, running, and rope skipping.

Walk

On the off chance that you can bear to go strolling, it will be an extraordinary method to battle a lot of weight. Now and then, you can choose to stroll to the accompanying store down the road as opposed to taking the vehicle. If you can require a couple of moments daily to walk a bit, it will assist you with accomplishing your objective of getting thinner. Think about a portion of these tips:

Take your dog for a walk each day

Consider pursuing cause strolls when conceivable Instead of taking the lift, use the stairwell.

A couple of meters to your home, get off the transport and walk the little distance to your home.

You can choose to leave your vehicle at the rear of the parcel and walk the leftover distance.

These are a portion of a couple of proposed methods of strolling. Wellness specialists accept that on the off chance that you can participate in a portion of these exercises for around 30 minutes every day, they will contribute fundamentally to your accomplishment in the fight against weight.

Change Your Sport

Incidentally, changing your game is another correct positive development on your approach to losing additional weight. On the off chance that you have gotten familiar with a specific game or exercise like lively strolling and others, you may consider adding different activities, for example, trekking to it. This is because your body gets acquainted with a game, the quantity of calories that your body consumes lessens.

The change may require your body to conform to move oxygen to every one of the tissues in your body. This can prompt expanded digestion, which will, at last, bring about extraordinary weight misfortune for you.

Lift Weights

Lifting weights is a characteristic technique for weight misfortune that is suggested by wellness specialists and a few people who are not, at this point, worried about their weights as they were before. Lifting weights will keep your body fit as a fiddle by assisting you with consuming amassed fats in the body. How? Siphoning iron expands the rate at which you consume calories while sitting. It additionally gives the body's digestion a decent lift by assisting it with consuming an overabundance of calories in the body quicker than the body will usually do. Attempt some push-ups, squats, and pull-ups and see the impact on your weight over the long run.

Continually Be in Motion

Try not to fail to understand the situation. The thought isn't that you ought to continually move, just start with one spot then onto the next. All things considered, that is incomprehensible. In any case, little demonstrations of development are powerful in consuming calories. Developments like extending, pacing, crossing, and uncrossing your legs are certain methods of decreasing weight.

As indicated by Mayo Clinic, a few groups were approached to eat additional 1000 calories every day for a very long time. Toward the finish of the two months, the individuals who continually squirmed didn't aggregate the calories as fat, while the individuals who were consistently fixed collected the calories. In this way, don't sit for long in a spot, pace when you are on the telephone or accomplishing something different.

Individuals love to sit in front of the TV a great deal. Individuals additionally need to appreciate great wellbeing, including having the correct weight. If the climate isn't helpful for an open-air workout, you can turn your TV to your wellspring of activity. You can check out wellness or weight misfortune station and exercise alongside them. On the off chance that you are watching a music station, you can move alongside them as opposed to watching them on your seat with your number one organic product juice in your grasp. The little exercise will add to your weight misfortune as you will actually want to consume a few calories all the while.

Figuring out how to Avoid Temptations and Triggers

While advising an individual to receive the characteristics of the intellectually solid is a decent method to create mental sturdiness, it may not generally be sufficient. As it were, it's somewhat similar to advising an individual that to be sound, you need to eat right, work out, and get a lot of rest. Such exhortation is acceptable and surprisingly right; notwithstanding, it does not have a specific particularity that can leave an individual inclination uncertain of precisely what to do. Luckily, a few practices can make an unmistakable arrangement of how to accomplish mental sturdiness. These practices resemble the real plans and activities expected to eat right and get a lot of activities. By embracing these practices into your day-by-day schedule, you will start to create mental strength in all that you do, and in each climate, you wind up in.

Stop Emotional Eating

The vast majority of us don't know we're passionate eaters, or we don't believe it's that serious. For a few of us, it doesn't prompt sensations of disgrace or weight acquire.

We can comfort a few of us and believe it is anything but a serious deal, yet it is.

Among others, passionate eating is out of equilibrium, something that can overwhelm our regular day-to-day existences. This may seem like overpowering longings or appetite; however, it's simply the inclination that we feel eager, powerless, and add to our weight.

Solace food gives us quick delight and removes the inclination.

Assimilation and sensation require a great deal of time, and the body can't do it.

Solace eating assists us with stifling agony since we flood our stomach-related plot with toxic waste.

At the point when we feel restless, feeling a major void opening inside us like we're eager can be normal. Rather than defying what this implies, i.e., our feelings, we're stuffing it down. In culture, it appears we are hesitant to feel an excess of that we don't realize we're running from our sentiments a large part of the time.

On the off chance that we don't allow ourselves to respond, we'll curb it. You will feel depleted until you start to allow yourself to feel the musings or sentiments that arise and abstain from stuffing down. It is because the body discharges past repressed feelings, and it can strike you hard.

That is the reason it tends to be difficult to relinquish passionate eating, as we need to vanquish the underlying "alarm" to proceed onward and begin figuring out how to acknowledge feelings for what they are. To be available, permitting an inclination to wash over us is magnificent and ought to be valued.

The more you permit yourself to be right now and feel, the fewer sentiments that overwhelm you, the less scared you will be. The passionate strength likewise diminishes. You'll turn out to be intellectually and truly more grounded.

At the point when it's off your stomach, you'll feel such a great deal better compared to supplanting it with food.

Getting to this point isn't quick. A few groups can part their passionate eating by better sustaining their bodies to dispose of actual longings and supporting others when they feel restless or enthusiastic.

To stop enthusiastic eating, you should be aware of how and why you eat, requiring a day out to consider what fulfills you. Numerous individuals don't see genuine yearning!

When you're eating intellectually, would you be able to stop yourself?

Could you sit and let the feeling wash over you as opposed to eating, allow yourself to feel it, and move it? Or then again, would you converse with somebody about how you feel?

Try not to harm yourself.

Passionate eating is normally something you've done since the beginning since it's essential for your make-up. It's a pursued routine, so you've figured out how to adapt to the climate.

It requires some investment to fix something so imbued in you, so if you wind up eating out of blame, if you jumble up, gain from it, and simply proceed onward. Acknowledgment is the initial step. If you realize you eat securely, you can overcome it.

Journaling will likewise assist you with perceiving dietary patterns. Note down previously, during, and after dinner. What caused eating was genuine yearning?

To figure out how to keep away from passionate eating, I can help. For quite a long time, I experienced an enthusiastic eating plague, here and there going on an everyday voraciously consuming food long-distance race. I never truly comprehended what caused these eating upheavals, all I knew was that I would begin eating and not stop until the food was gone, or anybody close to me saw me.

The circumstance rose, and my weight began to increment. Any eating routine I was on would in a split second, fall flat, and my fearlessness arrived at a record-breaking low. My eating causes were believed to be identified with work pressure, however, so numerous others may have an impact. Connections, wretchedness, monetary challenges, and numerous others will handily burn through gorge groupings.

At the point when I began attempting to sort out some way to keep away from passionate eating, I didn't have the foggiest idea where to begin. Like you, I went on the web and began examining. I went through the entire day perusing, processing and assembling passionate fix information, at that point around 3 a.m. I discovered my hero that morning.

Chapter 4 - Hypnosis For Weight Loss

At the point when it includes getting into shape, you have confidence in the quality go-to specialists: subject matter experts, nutritionists, and dietitians, wellness mentors, even passionate health tutors. Regardless, there could be the one you haven't definitely considered at this point: a subconscious subject matter expert.

It appears using hypnosis is another road people are meandering down for the purpose of weight loss. Moreover, generally, it's pursued the differed frantic endeavors (I see you, juice cleanses and pattern eats less) are endeavored and failed, says Greg Gurniak, an authorized clinical and clinical subconscious expert practicing in Ontario.

Regardless, it isn't about someone else controlling your brain and making you attempt savvy things while you're negligent. "Mind control and letting completely go, in any case, alluded to as achieving something without needing to, and are the best-misinformed decisions about hypnosis," says Kimberly Friedmutter. She is a daze-trained professional and maker of Subconscious Power: Use Your Inner Mind to cause the Life You Always Wanted. "Given how news sources portray daze inducers, people are lightened to find out I'm not wearing a dull robe and swinging a watch from a succession."

This substance is imported from {embed-name}. You would conceivably have the decision to find an indistinguishable significance in another arrangement; else, you may require the choice to get more information at their site.

You're also not absent once you experience hypnosis, it's all the more practically like an underground administration of loosening up, Friedmutter explains.

"It's basically the customary, floaty tendency you get before you nod off to rest or that brilliant sensation you are feeling as you ascend in the initial segment of the earlier day you're totally aware of where you're and what's incorporating you."

Being in that state makes you be all the more exposed to differ, which is the reason hypnosis for weight loss could be fruitful. "It's unique concerning various procedures since hypnosis keeps an eye on the reasoning and other contributing parts straightforwardly at the inward psyche level in the person's mind. Where their memories, inclinations, fears, food affiliations, negative self-talk, and certainty develop," says Capri Cruz, Ph.D., psychotherapist, and daze inducer and maker of Maximize Your Super Powers. "No other weight loss method keeps an eye on the central issues at the premise as hypnosis does."

Does Hypnosis Work for Weight Loss Work?

There is anything but a tremendous measure of later, randomized investigation available in regards to the matter, yet what's out there suggests that the strategy may be possible. Early examinations from the 90s found that people who used hypnosis lost double the greatest measure of weight as the individuals who consumed fewer calories without scholarly treatment. A new report worked with 60 rotund ladies and found that the people who practiced Hypno social treatment shed pounds and improved their dietary examples and self-discernment. Besides, a little 2017 examination worked with eight major adults and three children, every one of whom successfully shed pounds, with one, regardless, avoiding system because of the treatment benefits; none of this is frequently conclusive.

"The offensive factor is that hypnosis isn't instantly gotten by clinical insurance, so there's not an indistinguishable push for hypnosis peruses as there's for drug ones," Dr. Cruz says. Be that since it might, with the always extending cost of doctor-supported medications, broad courses of action of possible indications. Therefore, the push for more ordinary different alternatives, Cruz is certain hypnosis will before long get more thought and assessment as a reasonable weight-loss approach.

Who Should Attempt Hypnosis for Weight Loss?

"The ideal contender is, really, an individual who encounters trouble clinging to a sound eating regimen and exercise program since they can't shake their negative inclinations," Gurniak says. "Slowing down call at dangerous affinities: like eating the whole sack of potato chips as against stopping when you're full, is an indication of a subconscious issue," he says.

"Your mind is that where your sentiments, penchants, and addictions are discovered," Friedmutter says. Besides, in light of the fact that hypnotherapy tends to the internal brain, instead of simply the insightful, it very well may be really convincing. In reality, an assessment examination from 1970 found hypnosis to have a 93% accomplishment rate, with fewer gatherings needed than both psychotherapy and lead treatment. "This convinced, for developing penchants, thought models, and direct, hypnosis was the most straightforward procedure," Friedmutter says.

Hypnotherapy doesn't need to be used on their forlorn, by the same token. Gurniak says, "Hypnosis can in like manner be used as an acclamation to other weight loss programs arranged by specialists to treat diverse prosperity conditions, be it diabetes, beefiness, joint agony, or cardiovascular ailment."

What's in store In a Treatment?

Gatherings can vary long, and therefore the framework is depending upon the master.

For instance, Dr. Cruz says her meetings usually last some place in the scope of 45, and 60 minutes; however, Fried mutter sees weight loss patients for 3 to four hours. Be that as it may, generally speaking, you'll desire to line down, loosen up along with your eyes shut, and let the daze inducer oversee you through explicit techniques and proposition, which will assist you with showing up your targets.

"The musing is to put together the mind to progress toward what sound and away has upheld what's unfortunate," Friedmutter says. "Through client history, I'm ready to choose subconscious hitches that sent the client off their remarkable outline of [health]. Much an identical as we discover the best approach to individuals handle our bodies with food, and we will discover the best approach to regard them."

Possibly you do see this model on TV: A performer, a self-declared daze subject matter expert, stays in front of a group of people, arms open, and invites people from the pack to go close by him at the center of consideration.

The daze expert at that point takes a watch and progressively falters it before the volunteers' eyes. "Tired... You're getting v-e-r-y lazy," he says. Minutes after the very actuality, he snaps his fingers, one individual starting crying kind of a canine. Snap! Another opening was loosening her pants.

The pack laughs because the social occasion in front of a group of people gets sillier and sillier.

This reality is frequently the speculation of hypnosis, which is that the justification using it for something as real as weight loss would sound incredible. Be that since it might, through and through trustworthiness, various people have looked out to daze experts to help them change their relationship to food and wellbeing. Furthermore, various people have found phenomenal accomplishments.

It makes one marvel: This technique is motivated by a clinical master, practically like an advisor or trained professional. Does it show up as though what we see in front of a group of people?

"People regularly puzzle hypnotherapy with stage hypnosis for entertainment, and truly, the two have basically no to attempt to with each other," says Samantha Gaies, Ph.D., an authorized clinical clinician at NY Health Hypnosis and Integrative Therapy. Also, she works with individuals that had the chance to get better or recover from dietary issues. This is what the issue here is, and how it can help you in improving your way of life.

How Clinical Hypnosis Work?

At the point when someone is endeavoring to carry out a critical improvement in their life, such as overcoming heftiness, there is regularly a great arrangement to consider: what sustenances you need to eat, how you should register, and where you will have a method of safety enough to work out, for instance. Singular choices or fears may obstruct outlining day's end inclinations that would change an individual's prosperity.

"I, generally speaking, portray hypnosis to my patients by contrasting their current characters with a hamster wheel," says Dr. Gaies. "There's a consistent turn of events or thinking, yet that thinking doesn't regularly get them uncommonly far when it includes carrying out huge upgrades."

Subsequently, clinical subconscious experts hope to control their patients into a spur-of-the-moment state, in fact, called a surprise, using different strategies that change from significant breathing to insight.

As against standard reasoning, a surprise will not make them stroll around very much like the Walking Dead. Surely, the more critical a piece of us enters a daze once we are gazing vacantly at nothing in particular or doing a standard task. Our "hamster mind" stops pivoting these occasions, and that we died down fixated on our arrangement for the day or ordinary stressors. Once in that surprised state, Dr. Gaies strolls her patients through exercises to assist them with matured top of their needs to fluctuate.

In hypnosis, you're really endeavoring to drive the frontal cortex to make changes. "Hypnosis is fruitful because it grants people the possibility to obstruct the indicative and academic babble in their minds to all or any the more adequately access, and focus on what's more significant down and typically basic to them," says Dr. Gaies.

Thusly, hypnosis can help people with exploiting their internal brain frontal cortex, which, to a brilliant degree, impacts our penchants.

"The mind is that the spot a lot of our practices and motivations are," says Tony Chon, M.D., an authorized daze subject matter expert and a general internal specialist at the Mayo Clinic in Rochester, MN. "In hypnosis, you're really endeavoring to impact the psyche to make changes."

Chapter 5 - Training Your Brain to Burn Fat Fast

Burn fat fast and train your brain with this guide to finding your perfect workout.

Losing weight is rarely a quick process, but it can be relatively easy when you know where to start (and how to stay motivated). In fact, there are many different methods for burning fat, and if you find the right one for you, success will be as close as the next workout session.

The most essential thing about any training program is consistency, but that's not all. You should also make sure it's time-efficient, enjoyable, doesn't invoke any negative side effects (e.g., if a fitness plan doesn't fit into your life), and matches your goals (e.g., if you're a runner, your plan shouldn't be based on weightlifting). In this post, we'll look into how to identify what kind of workouts will keep you consistent.

So let's get started.

1.   **Identify your ultimate goal:** If you're not sure what your ultimate goal is, it can be easy to forget why you're working out in the first place. Your goal could be losing 20 pounds, running your first marathon, or just getting some extra energy. Whatever it is, make sure that the purpose of your workouts always stays clear and present in your mind.

2.   **Identify your training type:** If you're confused about whether you should be doing high-intensity interval workouts or long slow distance (LSD) workouts or something else because the workout is effective for most people, I usually suggest you choose a combination of both options.

For example, if you're a runner and want to lose weight, I would recommend doing some LSD training and high-intensity interval training.

3. **Keep your goals in mind:** While doing intense strength training won't necessarily help you lose weight (especially if performed too frequently), it's important to make sure that you still stay focused on your ultimate goal. For example, if you're running your first marathon, it would be counter-productive to train too hard. Instead, focus on building up endurance and speed instead.

4. **Remove distractions:** It's important to make sure that your goals stay clear and present in your mind while you're working out. However, that doesn't mean that you should be short-circuiting all forms of distractions while working out (as this can lead to burnout). At the same time, it's also true that you should avoid adding unnecessary stressors into your life when trying to lose weight.

5. **Stay within your limits:** On the other hand, it's also important to make sure that you're not pushing yourself too hard. While intensity is great for your progress, it's better to start off slow and gradually build up your strength over time.

6. **Make workouts a priority:** If you want to lose weight, you need to accept that exercise is something you'll be doing for the next few months or even years (depending on how long it'll take you to reach your ultimate goal). So, if you keep scheduling a lot of social activities for the same time as your workout session (e.g., because you like spending time with friends), then it might not be worth going through with the actual workout session.

7. **Speak to a trainer:** If you're not sure how much weight you should be lifting, how many calories you should be burning, or what type

of diet is best for you, then it makes sense to speak to a professional before making any diet or exercise decisions. Even if a personal trainer costs money, it's worth the investment because it eliminates many of the risks and complications associated with the process.

8.   **Get your training gear:** Finally, even if you decide that working out without equipment isn't for you (and it might not be), you'll still benefit from getting yourself some high-quality weights and a set of kettlebells to use at home. This will allow you to get a full workout session in at any time, which is especially useful if you're only doing workouts every few days (e.g., because of work or school commitments).

If you can follow these 8 simple rules, you'll be using your workout sessions to burn fat and get healthier for life. Now that's something I can get behind!

Chapter 6 - Visualization For Weight Loss

One of the biggest difficulties in shedding pounds is getting your psyche adjusted along with your objectives. Your brain is typically lined up with what you DON'T need, detrimental routines, lethargy, keeping away from exercise, and reckless activities, everything being equal.

Shedding pounds is extreme under those conditions, if not completely inconceivable.

You're continually taking on an internal conflict at whatever point you might want to pick between eating and exercise.

You want to make the most straightforward moves to get in shape and accomplish your objectives, however, you may don't have any desire to make those moves on account of the best tons more effort than taking the immediate way and remaining along with your old propensities.

One of the foremost viable procedures for overcoming any barrier among psyche and body is visualization.

Visualization can help you to shed pounds in 2 essential manners:

First, it can help you to beat those inward boundaries we just covered.

On the off chance that you are doing it right, changing your propensities will appear to be practically effortless.

You'll get in shape the probability of self-damage and think that it's a lot simpler to embrace sound propensities and stick with them all the time.

Second, visualization is frequently staggeringly propelling.

One of the primary reasons individuals hand over their solid eating regimen and exercise plan is to become weary of it. They get uninterested in eating comparable old food sources for a long time; they get uninterested in doing identical exercises for quite a while and lose interest.

Visualization might be a fantastic antitoxin for low inspiration. It's perhaps the easiest approach to restore your inspiration consistently and keep it continuing forward, all gratitude to your objective.

Visualization additionally can be utilized for loads of different objectives you'll have other than weight loss. It's a hearty instrument regularly utilized by money managers, competitors, big names, and fruitful individuals from varying backgrounds.

We're having the chance to have some expertise in the weight loss application in this guide, yet keep in mind that you basically can, without much of a stretch, utilize an identical cycle for any objective you'll be pursuing, presently or later on.

What Is Visualization?

Visualization is the way toward seeing pictures to you.

For instance, if I requested that you accept a dawn, you'd likely see a quick picture of the sun ascending into the great beyond. If I requested that you think about an apple, you'd see it intellectually somewhat like you saw the dawn.

In case you're similar to the vast majority, you didn't have a drag "seeing" this stuff intellectually.

Notwithstanding, a few groups struggle imagining pictures. They will accept many different items, yet they don't actually "see" them intellectually.

If that is your experience as well, don't stress over it. In all honesty, you don't have to see pictures intellectually to utilize visualization adequately.

I'm having the chance to share another tip that will help you to utilize visualization regardless of if you'll see mental pictures.

Utilizing Visualization for Weight Loss

To utilize visualization for weight loss, you only made little "mental films" about circumstances that you need to make right. Underneath, we'll reexamine some of the foremost regular approaches to utilize visualization for weight loss.

Before we do this present, it's crucial to notice that visualization will be undeniably more powerful in case you're setting aside the effort to get extremely loosened up first. Feeling focused or tired will make it harder for you to think, and your visualization meetings will not be close to as functional.

To get loose, take 5 to 10 minutes to sit down discreetly and discharge strain from your psyche and body. Inhale profoundly and gradually, envisioning that you are just delivering tension and stress with each exhalation.

Zero in on each muscle bunch in your body and let it unwind, each in turn. You'll even picture the muscles gradually giving up, getting agreeable, limp, and loose. At the point when you feel completely loose and quiet, at that point you'll begin with one of the visualization procedures underneath:

Envisioning the End Result

The most widely recognized use for visualization is seeing the "result" of the objective you're attempting to achieve. For weight loss purposes, you'd have some expertise in a picture of yourself, weighing what you might want to consider and wearing the measurements and style of attire you might want to wear.

You may envision yourself in a specific setting that you do been anticipating, similar to your secondary school gathering, a family wedding, or just relaxing on the sea shore in a bathing suit.

You can likewise make the visualization more dynamic by that work in an active work you're doing. For instance, you would perhaps see yourself running, swimming, fidgeting with your youngsters, or strolling, as it were, along with your head held high, overflowing with certainty each progression.

Incorporate however many subtleties in this vision as you like. What are you wearing?

How can one feel? What does your hair best like? Who is with you in the thought? What do your environmental factors best like? What do they possess an aroma like? How are the climate and temperature?

Zeroing in on these little subtleties can help make your visualization meetings undeniably more practical and, up to this point, all the more remarkable.

Stay with the vision however long you like, 10 minutes around is incredible, yet you'll abound in the feed for broadened on the off chance that you might want.

Attempt to make the vision so genuine and incredible that you feel like you're truly there, encountering it right away.

Visualization for Motivation

Getting roused with visualization is more straightforward than you would potentially think, and it doesn't take an all-encompassing effort to attempt to.

Start by getting extremely loose, and afterward, accept what it appears as though to be propelled. You positively encountered the impression of being inspired at some time or another, that sensation of being exceptionally invigorated and energized, needing to get breaking, and making a move now!

Zero in on that inclination, and picture feeling that route about your weight loss exercises. Envision feeling so roused and inspired that you basically can hardly wait to begin your exercises each day. Envision feeling so extraordinary after each activity that you're pleased you most likely did it. Envision anticipating getting ready good suppers and bites and feeling extraordinary because you're energizing your body with incredible nourishment.

In case you're prepared to tune into genuine sensations of inspiration in your visualization meeting, those sentiments will stay with you, particularly if you do this day by day.

You're having the opportunity to find that you are normally more persuaded about staying along with your solid way of life.

You'll program your psyche to believe that these activities are charming and comfortable, and your body will fit toward doing them normally. You will not have to drive yourself to attempt to do them any longer.

51

Visualization to Spice Up Your Workouts

If you at any point want to stay away from practice since it would seem that an unnecessary measure of work, this visualization practice helps you tremendously.

It's been logically demonstrated that imagining yourself performing actual work can improve your performance. Competitors move in the feed constantly!

They are going through their routine intellectually again and again, and their performance improves thus, similarly as though they had been truly rehearsing!

You can utilize this equivalent interaction to upgrade your exercises' adequacy and even persuade yourself to work call at the essential spot.

Like we just covered above, you'll imagine yourself feeling extraordinary about comprehension, which can persuade you to work out each day. Nonetheless, you'll likewise go through an exercise in your psyche and picture that you're getting more grounded, quicker, and more productive.

Once more, don't simply "see" this to you; endeavor to FEEL it in your body as you imagine it. Feel your muscles working even as they would in a genuine exercise. (Clearly, it will not feel exactly equivalent to a genuine exercise, yet you'll make it pretty reasonable on the off chance that you concentrate.)

See you lifting weights rapidly, building fit muscle. See yourself improving your cardiovascular wellness instantly and quickly, making your exercises feels simpler.

Picture this stuff a day, and before long, you'll see that they seem, by all accounts, to be occurring, your exercises are feeling simpler, and you're getting fitter quicker than you'd have by opposing activity.

Visualization to Create Confidence

A typical indication of being overweight is low fearlessness. Perhaps the most significant reason why a considerable lot of us need to get in shape is they'll feel surer. Being fit and thin would permit them to forestall feeling like they need to cover or feel humiliated about their bodies.

Is That a hearty Goal for You Too?

Utilizing visualization every day can begin assembling your certainty even before you arrive at your objective weight.

The visualization practice is basic; imagine you feeling sure, solid, and enabled. Envision what it may want to be persuaded.

Envision going to parties and other social capacities and not agonizing over what others think about you. Envision giggling, moving, and making some genuine memories.

Envision getting wearing the morning and knowing your best extraordinary. Envision how that may change your entire attitude. Envision how you'd interface with individuals at work, in your family, and with outsiders freely.

In those potential situations, envision yourself feeling totally confident. Tune into that inclination as acutely as you'll, and stay with it however long you'll (10 or quarter-hour is fantastic). You'll likewise apply this activity once you are in a public spot.

Whenever you're out some place, and you start to feel somewhat timid or humiliated, bring to mind the sure self you do been picturing.

Recollect how it feels to be certain, solid, and confident, at that point, bring a little smidgen of that pith into yourself any place you end up being at that point. You'll see that doing this smaller than usual exercise makes you feel better and simpler.

Chapter 7 - Hypnosis Session to Improve the Relation with Food

At the point when it includes interesting associations, the direction can regularly make a step back or break; in any case, that is not, for the most part, another with food. We, all in all, will eat. In any case, for those people who have a fierce relationship with food, fundamental tasks like food shopping, eating out, or, regardless, picking what to cook at home can want a minefield.

As demonstrated by the bits of knowledge, we have seen a 24% development in stoutness-related clinical facility certifications in the U.K. over the late years. More than a third (35%) of adults in England are overweight, with an extra 28% being surveyed to fall under the fat order. Nonetheless, notwithstanding an interminable stream of government-moved designs to get us into week-by-week weight reduction classes and diets, doesn't work for big quantities of people. For what reason would that be, and is there a more possible way to deal with improve our relationship with what we eat?

Why Diets Work?

Restricting what we eat, following inflexible eating routine plans, or getting to week-by-week gatherings achieve explicit people's work. Nonetheless, this will frequently be a brief game plan that drives various to experience yo-yo slimming down, weight reduction, and weight acquire. Daze expert Becca Teers explains more.

"Diets won't come overall game plan with the enduring way of life changes needed, for example, a modest long stretch change in our dietary examples and attitude to food. Many eating routine plans are temporary and might be hard to keep up to date with an advancing reason, really because they're unreasonably restrictive or they prevent us from getting our favored sustenances."

So, while we may even see transient victories since we aren't trying our overall perspective on food, even as any secret issues which will have cause unwanted eating rehearses (for instance, using food as a route for taking care of pressure). We aren't setting ourselves up for the day's end accomplishment.

In reality, Becca explains, we may be making a more bad cycle for ourselves. "By making us count calories or intentionally measure solution size or perhaps totally reject kinds of sustenances, various eating regimens can make us more focused on food and our eating. This way will eliminate the joy from eating and lead us to long for a more noteworthy measure of explicit sustenances. An eating routine, gorge/gorge cycle can start."

Making us center around the probability that what we eat, and any connected weight stresses is basically the result of resolve. We had the chance to 'contribute more energy' to differ; diets can lead us to dismiss the fundamental issues that are really making us fight.

For What Reason Do I Battle with Food?

Dangerous relationship with food isn't 'just directly down to 'self-restraint.'

Tumultuous plans, points of view to food while growing up, and neglectful sentiments, feelings, or practices that we'd be clueless we've made would all be prepared to provoke unwanted relationships with food. Regardless of whether you fight with settling on more valuable food choices, reveling, or object to 'specific eating,' the odds are that there's a secret issue that you probably won't think about, or that you probably won't understand the best approach to fix. A portion of the basic reasons people can develop a bothersome relationship with food can include:

Comfort Eating

Otherwise called energetic, two or three individuals go for food to adjust to testing considerations, slants, sentiments, or conditions. On the off chance that you wrap up pursuing a chomp whenever you are vexed or centered around, use food as a way to deal with stir yourself to navigate an extraordinary task or rout weakness. These are altogether signs that you could likewise be using food as a way to deal with help your personality.

Stress

Perceiving the signs of strain is frequently serious. When we feel overwhelmed and unequipped for adjusting, it will in general, be a fair sign that we're under pressure. Regardless, two or three people, our sensations of craziness can consistently increase inevitably, and that we probably won't comprehend they're getting unmanageable as we intend to find ways to deal with self-fix to fluctuate how we are feeling.

We may even check whether our drinking augmentations as our sensations of insanity do.

Assume you start from a glass of wine to get over a disturbing day, up to 3, four, or possibly an entire container.

However, shouldn't something be said about what we eat? This way doesn't infer that each last lavishness is an indication of a more broad issue, yet food has its actual nature. As a whole appreciate reliably, we've to quantify what we can by trying to portray concerning plans.

Food Addictions

While there are still conversations enveloping the term 'food propensity,' many can concur that how we eat can fall into a sort of friendly impulse. Certain sustenances that will cause spikes in feel-incredible synthetic substances or our imperativeness levels can lead us to momentarily feeling unprecedented, yet regularly don't give us the interminable estimation of being full or satisfied. Inevitably, this will infer that we've to eat progressively a greater amount of something to get that identical tendency. This reality will incite further issues with slants of fault, shame, and may even oppositely influence your certainty and bravery.

Past Existence Encounters

Other fundamental factors from our pasts can influence our ceaseless points of view and practices around food. Past injury, abuse, taking in courses from our families, trouble adjusting to negative sentiments, torment, misfortune, or low certainty would contribute.

It Became a Propensity

Inevitably, negative personal conduct standards can make without our agreement. Perhaps you wrap up eating once you're not greedy; you, by and large, buy a snack together with your morning coffee; otherwise, you can't imagine going down the film without getting some popcorn. Distinguishing these inclinations on their desolate is frequently questionable.

Prosperity (Physical or Mental) Related Conditions

Hormonal unpredictable attributes, remedy results, and surprisingly certain mental prosperity conditions, similar to despairing or anxiety, would all be prepared to incite appalling eating practices or issues with food. In case you're worried that another central condition could be causing you eating issues, it is fundamental to talk together with your GP.

How Does Hypnotherapy Help?

Working with a subconscious expert can help you with watching out for a decent extent of issues and troubles. An experienced guide will decide to assist you with recognizing and address any principal reasons you would perhaps be engaging with food.

Hypnotherapy can help you discover how to deal with negative sentiments in a superior, sound, viable way, which will allow you to remain far away from solace eating. For the people who eat or snack without theory, for example, when you're getting ready or in suppers, if cautious eating doesn't work for you, gastric band hypnotherapy may require the decision to assist you with feeling full for additional. This way will help you with keeping away from bothersome sustenances.

Through working with a refined daze inducer, you'll learn new contraptions and methodology to assist you with regulating constant or fluctuating sensations of delirium, disquiet, or energetic over-trouble. With their help and course, you'll all the almost certain perceive how these could be affecting various parts of your life, beat all, assisting you with carrying out sure improvements which will have a more broad, constant impact.

As Julia shares through her comprehension of endeavoring hypnotherapy for exciting eating, hypnosis can help you discover how to talk with and fathom your body all the more promptly.

"It had gotten where I'd become focused [with food], and it wasn't uncommon for the benefit of me. I've gotten considerably less stressed over eating. I like it; notwithstanding, I've discovered how to eat when my body is greedy and not because my mind needs something to reduce my sentiments. Hypnotherapy has really assisted me with knowing things."

"I have started to get familiar with our inside models, where they begin from, and how we approach advancing them."

Hypnotherapy as a substitute for Treating Certain Addictions

A regular request when it includes hypnosis is: will it work for me? It's hard to comprehend until you endeavor it yourself. Studies have shown hypnotherapy is frequently a sound option for working with anxiety, treating certain addictions, and regardless, taking care of reveling.

Like a wide range of hypnotherapy, it requires a responsive standpoint, searching for a change, and responsibility. Two or three individuals may even see changes in the lead after only one gathering, while others may have a few gatherings to discover genuine overhauls. Your daze expert may introduce self-hypnosis techniques; you'll endeavor yourself between sessions to help with strengthening novel musings and backing progress.

Food is indispensable to life. We can outfit ourselves with imperativeness that impacts our disposition, even as how we see our bodies. We are, by and large exceptional, just like our eating regimens and ways of life. To be sound, for what it's worth, a steady relationship with food is basic.

Chapter 8 - Hypnosis Session to Stop Emotional Eating

You need gas food, similar to sustenance, and the staple to construct your cells, muscles, and cells. In any case, you more likely than not use nourishment for tons of reasons past those physiological prerequisites. Undoubtedly, food goes to be the highlight of a genuine article of your esteemed parties. Also, you would potentially utilize food as a quick and direct approach to feeling much improved on the off chance that you are feeling. Maybe you'll blend food affectionately, mindful, warm, sustaining, and family, in any event at a psyche level.

Denying yourself totally the wonderful feelings and social advantages that food can give is counterproductive later on. My estimate is you're thinking about being lean and glad, more slender, and hopeless. That is the explanation I'm not having the chance to request you all together to surrender any from your #1 food varieties or become a weirdo. It's significant to allow yourself satisfactory mercy not to feel denied; nonetheless, you might want adequate consistency to get the outcomes you need.

Carrying out dinners for nonphysical intentions turns into a drag on the off chance that you are doing it as how to deal with pressure or opposite thoughts, and you are doing it as often as possible or maybe unwittingly. A few specialists cause the topic of mental eating to show up so profound; you'd trust it may require many years of intervention to beat. I really don't think emotional eating is muddled at all. It is a direct issue rotating around three fundamental topics:

- You do and undetectably, without accepting.

- You eat for reasons other than physiological necessities.

- You do have confidence in food varieties that don't propel you toward your points.

The center of the condition is that you once in a while eat for some unacceptable reasons, and you would perhaps not remember it.

Why You Eat When you are not Physically Hungry

Numerous ladies and men misjudge that emotional eating just occurs in light of stress and deal with negative feelings like sorrow, despondency, despairing, or despair. Notwithstanding, individuals eat for a few distinct intentions that don't have anything to do with physiological requests, for instance:

- To lighten the pressure.

- To mingle

- To reproduce a sense or memory

- To notice a particular occasion

- To satisfy a vacancy or lacking need

- To feel better; to feel secured; to feel vulnerable; People eat as an advantage, out of convention or reliance (sleep time nibbling and eating before the TV).

Now and again, eating for nonphysical reasons is worthy, particularly for family social affairs, weddings, birthday celebrations, or occasions. You'll even convincingly affirm its privilege not to get included, particularly family and get-togethers, to the food that matches together.

62

Step-by-step instructions to Tell the Difference Between Physical and Emotional Hunger?

There are some exceptionally particular contrasts between mental and actual cravings.

Actual craving develops step by step, beginning with a little protest in the gut, creating extravagant cravings for food.

1.   Emotional craving develops abruptly.

2.   With actual hunger, it's probably going to join if you do too.

3.   Emotional hunger appears to request quick satisfaction.

4.   Actual craving often shows up around three hours following the supper or drink.

5.   Emotional hunger now and then happens whenever.

6.   Actual yearning is regularly an overall hunger for dinners.

7.   Emotional craving is regularly a prerequisite for a chose dinner.

8.   After ingestion for actual craving, the hunger disappears.

9.   After emotional ingestion, the hunger proceeds.

10.   After ingestion for actual craving, you get a method of fulfillment.

11.   After eating for emotional reasons, you are feeling remorseful.

The Truth About Physical Hunger and Dietary

Restriction

A ton of dietitians and therapists encourage you should eat in case you're eager.

If their objective is that you basically need to feast because of genuine actual longing, not emotional need, I concur. Nonetheless, on the off chance that you decipher this as "Consistently devour at whatever point you're not kidding," that I really don't feel that it's amazing counsel. Suppose you do satisfy your calorie recompense each day; notwithstanding, you are as yet wiped out hungry?

In case you might want to get slimmer, you settle on a caloric deficiency, which as a rule, implies you will be eager once in a while. If you answer every sensation of physiological craving for a little to eat, you'll drop your caloric shortfall. I'm not discussing starvation slims down that produce wild cravings. I'm going to keep a little calorie deficiency, tolerating only tons of irregular hunger, and acquiring any dietary restriction.

It's difficult to excuse the genuine actual thirst experienced under dry season conditions since this state is the most cliché individual drive, significantly more masculine than simple proliferation.

Milestone research on starvation ran by Ancel Keys at the University of Minnesota numerous many years prior uncovered when subjects were devoured a semi-starvation diet at 50% of their upkeep caloric admission for a half-hour. Thusly, close by, the push to eat, turned out to be harsher and more difficult.

The subjects couldn't accept anything besides food. They lost interest in sex. It bodes well from an endurance viewpoint since in case you're ravenous and couldn't take care of, and you'd have the ability to endure and sustain sexes. In adolescence, hunger chemicals precisely develop while sex regenerative and drive capacities to fall. On low-carbohydrates slims down in inadequate muscle to fat ratio levels, ladies' cycle stopped, and men's testosterone levels dropped.

It causes a specific circumstance for forestalling outrageous low-carb to consume fewer calories as you will not at any point be in a situation to oppose the basic longing to get inconclusively. It's practically similar to rest. You'll deny yourself for simply a period, for an extreme price to your wellbeing, yet you can't fight the temptation. On the other side, any individual who discloses to you that accomplishing and keeping up your optimal weight doesn't best any dietary limitation has been one-sided. You do get aware of your body's signs and decide the best approach to respond suitably to them.

This reality will recommend not devouring, regardless of whether you truly want it. An incredible illustration of dietary limitation is frequently known among the Okinawans, among the least fatty and longest-lived occupants around Earth.

The class incorporates a legacy alluded to as Hari Hachi Bu, signifying, "Eat until you're just 80% complete." Compare that with the Western social propensity for "cleaning your plate" and "not wasting food varieties," and that we may have a reaction to why there's a heftiness emergency in the USA now.

Stop "Squandering" Your Food

In the long periods of social molding on your folks and culture, you'll have built up an idea you do to wash all the food off your plate, but you are as yet eager or not. You'll be customized to trust it's offensive to your host never to eat anything you're served so that it's disposed of cash if you don't eat whatever you do pay not to squander food if there are less honored people on Earth who are eager.

May I recommend a specific point of view? On the off chance that you keep eating after you're as of now full, you're squandering food in any case since totality might be a fairly solid sign your energy needs are met. You needn't bother with that caloric energy; thus, the overabundance gets stored as fat. What's more, that is a genuine "squander." Incidentally, in case you're in a situation to bring up to me that cleaning up what plate may help starving youngsters in Africa, at that point, let me see precisely how it helps, and that I will go along with you.

Recall that one among the principal win convictions of helpless people is transparency. We don't perform "living in fantasy land" in the Body Fat Remedy application, we perform exact reasoning, and we are set up to have a go at doing anything significant. Just a little craving ought to be expected as you're at a calorie deficiency, and it's a neighborhood of the worth that you essentially purchase getting more slender.

Neglectfully you are doing not wish to eat at whatever point you're ravenous. Just because you'd prefer to devour doesn't really imply that you just ought to.

If you fear to crave, you'll routinely eat to have around the inclination.

You'll comprehend the best approach to suffer hunger. Advise yourself that there are examples in your day-to-day existence when you do been eager and stayed. You will endure because thirst isn't ever an emergency.

Another approach to appear to be after want is to utilize your new abilities. On the off chance that a calorie shortage causes fat cells, assuming a little craving includes a calorie deficiency, why not change your assessment: "It isn't hunger; it is the inclination of fat cells."

The A.W.A.R.E. Recipe: Five Steps Which End

Emotional Eating

Mindfulness is that the beginning line of shift can't handle a drag in the event that you don't have any acquaintance with yourself. You will discover how to make a sharp Comprehension of your standards of conduct, the best approach to stop unwanted Designs inert in their courses, likewise as the best approach to substitute them with new ones. You'll likewise have to realize how to roll out the improvements perpetual using your sensory system; thusly, the negative examples aren't probably going to happen. Positive new eating practices will work on autopilot.

There are five straightforward activities for this interaction, which I conjecture, the A.W.A.R.E. recipe:

- Be mindful of your eating practices.

- Be cautious about mental eating triggers.

- Arrest the personal conduct standards at whatever point they occur.

- Replace the old mental eating conduct with substantially more compelling decisions.

- Establish pristine convictions about food and furthermore the correct explanations behind ingestion.

Chapter 9 - Hypnosis Session for Perfect Portion Control

Section control can accept a major part in achieving your prosperity and weight goals. You may, as of now, be eating many sustenances and taking fitting action.

In any case, if you wrap up passing on excess weight, it very well may be because you're simply using unreasonably. Part control can have a serious impact.

Extraordinary part control will not simply aim you to slimmer, it gives you greater essentialness. Eating the correct total will mean your body truly should try to handle an unnecessary wealth of food.

Part Control Is About the Right Measure of Food

The sum is pretty much as critical as quality when it includes getting your eating routine right and shedding excess fat. An excess of something that is generally acceptable really is frequently horrible for you once you need to get fit as a fiddle.

Nonetheless, it can feel hard to see how, when, and therefore the sum to chop down with the objective that you can really begin to discover some improvement in showing up at your weight goals.

For what reason is it so difficult to practice parcel control?

Penchant drives our continues with significantly more than we comprehend.

We eat because it's a perfect chance to eat (regardless of the very truth that you essentially had a snack just thirty minutes back). We enjoy out of obligingness, or not wanting to 'waste' what's on our plate, or because we are stuffing ourselves that we've ignored the best approach to see when we've had enough.

Some sensible things will help you with controlling part size:

• You can intentionally eat all the more step by step; this permits your stomach to enroll its entirety in your brain and cut your hankering.

• You regularly gin your supper with soup, a low-calorie soup can be satisfying and grant you to feel content with tons smaller fragments for your standard course.

• You can use the old, more diminutive plate stunt, so you genuinely had the opportunity to eat tinier fragments.

• You can keep an essential separation from smorgasbords and disregard 'uber feast' deals.

Why Hypnosis Is an Integral Asset for Part Control Astonishing

Based on the total of the above admonishment could likewise be, you truly had the chance to overcome affinity and drive, and that is where hypnosis can really help. Food is fuel, and fuel ought to be of the correct quality and sum. Imagine endeavoring to place more fuel into your vehicle when it's full.

It just doesn't look good.

The Portion Control hypnosis meeting will bring you into a significantly extricated state and quickly train your careless brain to normally ignore bounty food and license your absorption to be an astounding arrangement more pleasant. You'll rediscover the pleasure of being on top of your body prerequisites for food.

Why is Part Control troublesome?

Our inclinations rule our lives, we eat for a couple of quantities of reasons than required. We eat:

- Because high sugar and sodium "welcome" us to attempt to naturally, satisfying our necessity for extra.
- Because we know about stuffing ourselves.
- Out of benevolence.
- Not wanting to waste.
- Because we've neglected what sum is adequate.
- Because we are depleted, debilitate, or furious.

Part Control Assumes a Big Function in Your Life

You, as of now, could be eating many sustenances and managing out.

Notwithstanding, on the off chance that you wind up passing on extra weight or pounds that just will not shed, it will be the situation that you only are basically consuming unreasonably. Portion control includes a huge impact.

Right Segment Control influences your vitality and digestion controlling your pieces when eating doesn't only motivate you to slimmer; similarly, it's a trigger part in your body that gives you greater essentialness and assembles your processing. At the point when the body has more food "threw at it," your body should endeavor to measure and ingest unnecessary food. This way takes extra imperativeness and makes your processing deferred as your body sets up a careful instrument.

Weight reduction Hypnosis Included on Morning America

Incredible Morning America incorporated a lady who shed 140 pounds and kept it off for a long time. See how she changed her desires from modest food to strong sustenances. She went from 287 to 147 pounds. Snap here to notice the hypnosis for weight reduction report on morning America.

Beat Propensity and Impulse Issues with Hypnosis for Part Control

You need to beat the affinity and drive drew in with segment control issues, which is that the spot hypnosis might be an amazing mechanical assembly.

Hypnosis for parcel control brings you into a significantly relaxed up mode. It retrains your mind-brain to naturally forsake the excess of food, allowing your processing to augment because a savvy proportion of food is being given to the body. Rediscover the fulfillment in being on top of your body, and without that abnormal, powerful tendency after you eat and "it happened again… I gorged."

See what hypnosis can essentially mean for the heading of your life.

Become progressively more focused on your targets, acquire, appreciate a more unmistakable slant of confidence and satisfaction, and see more results from your headway, it's all possible with hypnosis.

Hypnosis Is Demonstrated More Successful Than Talk Treatments

In an examination in American Health Magazine, hypnosis and hypnotherapy have a 93% accomplishment rate. Interestingly with lower results from various treatment methods, which best obviously more gatherings?

Snap here to get familiar with hypnosis and its high accomplishment rate.

You're Prepared to Utilize Hypnosis as a Useful Asset for Sound Part Control

Affinities rule our lives and shape our current reality; in any case, it moreover shapes our future presence. Portion control is presumably the foremost convincing inspiration for why people are set on weight. Indeed, although it's not sound acceptable for two or three, it will address your weight reduction adventure's choosing the second.

In hypnotherapy, you might want to control your brain, which can allow you to deal with your penchants and tendencies you do rapidly. There are various reasons why people gorge. Some probably won't say that people pick the choice to attempt to in this way, which implies it's moreover seen as unmindful eating.

Bit by Bit Instructions to Beat Portion Control and Overeating Difficulties

We need food to suffer; notwithstanding, when does it take food shows up at some degree where it achieves reveling? When it is vital to look at you, take a step back, and quit eating?

Every person who has an unfortunate relationship with food sees it in like manner. It regularly fills in as a comfort and security technique that permits us to impact ourselves that it's able exhausts food thoughtlessly and without allowance. Clearly, aside from in case you're set up in food or worth agonizing about your flourishing, you probably don't have a positive relationship with food.

Change Your Eating Habits

Assume you do see the need to build a prevalent relationship with food. You would conceivably need to search out additional about hypnosis for weight reduction and kick your negative standards of conduct. In all things considered, you might want to detect the hidden explanation adding to your anxiety. Since eating presents itself as a sort of transient pressing factor easing and redirects us from feeling sentiments like pressing factor, pity, disquiet and shock, it's something we watch out for slant toward at any rate in the long run in our lives. However long advancing associations are experts at giving blemished society sustenances that will give off an impression of being connecting with or are peddled into a point "dietary-obliging" content, we've accepted the conviction that it's okay to exhaust fake food or whatever publicizing prescribes to us.

We've correspondingly educated ourselves that spending unfortunate food goes about like a prize for whatever we're progressing admirably.

Make an effort not to Punish Yourself

For instance, uncovering to yourself that you can eat anything you want all through the highest point of the week following five non-end of the week-long periods of unpolluted eating is altogether misguided. We should not feel like we are rebuking ourselves by eating a strong, changed eating

74

regimen. It should wind up being normal to us as we get a sound way of life.

The underlying advance to using hypnosis for compelling weight reduction is recognizing the clarifications of why you fight to achieve whatever it's you might want. When perusing self-hypnosis, you should discover how to address your food obsession and transform it into something significant, for example, motivation to not feel however feeble or inefficient as you may be doing at your present weight state of prosperity. Before you start, you need to perceive the inspiration driving why your goal seems, by all accounts, to be hitherto off, even as the thing it's that is keeping you far away from achieving it.

What Will the Hypnotherapy Session Be Like?

In a specialist hypnotherapy meeting, an expert will, for the foremost part, ask you an overview of requests related to weight reduction, including questions concerning your eating regimen and exercise inclinations. Since you're coordinating the therapy meeting all alone, you'll reconsider your step-by-step timetable and penchants. Now and again, it helps record your positive and negative propensities to find out where you do to improve. You do to format everything of the information before you and spotlight what you need to improve in your gathering. Recording your destinations will in like manner, help you develop a clearer picture of where you'd like better to go. Recall that self-hypnosis is absolutely dependent upon you, so you might want to submit and stay prepared in the 21 days.

Chapter 10 - Building Motivation

Motivation is one of the principal integral assets in making perpetual change. Your explanation is predicated on your opinion. Furthermore, as you're presumably mindful, conviction is hardly upheld by your solid reality. Generally, you think things because of how you see them, believe them, hear them, and smell them, at that point forward. You'll program your psyche by taking sentiments from one among your encounters and interfacing those sentiments to an exceptional event. Permit us to look at how you'll stay inspired to get thinner:

Start Where You're Now

You should take a full-length image of yourself at this as a push system from your present position. Two essential variables apply to wellbeing. One is whether you wish the picture you find in the mirror, and consequently, the second is how you feel. Do you have the energy to attempt to do what you might want, and would you say you are feeling sufficient?

Investigate your purposes behind anxiety to get more fit. These are the thing will keep you going even once you don't want it.

Evaluate your dietary patterns and set up your explanations behind gorging or enjoying some unacceptable food varieties. It is accepted that you just have the will to get better and get more fit.

Here, you state plainly and emphatically to yourself what you might want, and afterward conclude that you essentially will achieve it with industriousness. Utilize the self-entrancing routine disclosed above to crash now into your inner mind.

Decide your motivation for the predefined results and how you'll know when you do achieve the objective. How might you feel, what you'll see, and what you are probably going to tune in to once you accomplish your objective?

Dedicate the initial meeting of self-entrancing to making the final word choice about your weight. Note that you essentially should not at any point have any uncertainty in your brain about your test to get more fit.

Plan your suppers daily. Gauge yourself oftentimes to watch your advancement too. Notwithstanding, don't be distrustful about gauging yourself, as this will contrarily influence your advancement.

Rehash to yourself daily that you just are turning out to be to your optimal weight, that you do grow new, reasonable dietary patterns, which you're not helpless to allurement.

Think decidedly and supply positive insistences in your self-prompted mesmerizing state.

Change Your Lifestyle

Each seemingly insignificant detail checks. This sentence is frequently urgent to see on the off chance that you might want to get thinner and shed pounds. Several progressions in your normal day-by-day exercises can help you to consume more calories.

Walk More

Utilize the means instead of the lift in case you're simply rising or down a story or two.

Park your vehicle a mile far away from your objective and walk the rest of the way. You'll likewise walk energetically to consume more calories.

Make it more dynamic in your day of rest by taking your canine for an all-encompassing stroll in the recreation center.

If you might want to a few squares, save gas and keep away from traffic by strolling. For more noteworthy distances, dust off that old bicycle and pedal your way to your objective.

Watch How and What You Eat

A major breakfast kicks your body into hyper-digestion mode, so you should not skirt the essential feast of the day.

Brushing after a dinner flags your brain to get done with eating, causing you to want less until your next booked supper.

On the off chance that you might want to get food from a café, make your request to-go so you will not get enticed by their different contributions.

Plan your suppers for the week, so you'll check which level of calories you're devouring in a day.

Make fast, quality dinners, so you save time. There are a large number of plans out there. Do some examination.

Eat at a table, not in your vehicle. Drive-through food is almost consistently oily and loaded up with undesirable crabs.

Put more leaves, similar to arugula and horse feed sprouts on your dinners to offer you more fiber and cause you to eat less.

Request the smallest dinner size if you had the opportunity to eat nutriment.

Start your feast with a vegetable plate of mixed greens. Dunk the plate of mixed greens into the dressing as opposed to pouring it on.

For a light in-between meal, crunch on protein bars, or basically drink a glass of skimmed milk.

Eat before you go to the staple to hold yourself back from being enticed by food things you don't choose to purchase.

Wipe out your storeroom by eliminating foods that will not help you along with your wellness objectives.

The entire thought in the changes referenced is that you basically ought to eat less and move more. You'll be prepared to think about extra changes. Show them down close by those found in this book.

The Power of Affirmations

Today is basically one more day. Today might be a day for you to begin making a euphoric, satisfying life. Presently it's your day to start to deliver every one of your hindrances. Presently your day allows you to get private the favored experiences of life. You'll change yourself into an improving issue. You, presently, incorporate the contraption inside one to perform naturally. These gadgets are accurately your interests and your feelings.

What Are Positive Affirmations?

I may wish to explain a little pretty much each one of those that aren't familiar with the upsides of positive confirmations. A public statement is whatever you say or, all things being equal, think. An unfathomable arrangement of what we by and large report and feel are somewhat risky. It doesn't have incredible encounters for us. We'll retain our support and furthermore to talk into positive models on the off chance that we'd prefer to change us totally.

It's a starting point on the least complex approach to adjusting. Customarily, you're saying to your psyche head: "I'm accepting obligation. I'm careful that there is something that I can do to change" While I talk about doing certifications, I propose deliberately choosing words that will either help take something out from your Life or make something new in your life. Every thought you think, and each word you say is a confirmation, everything of oneself talk, our inside market, perhaps a surge of promises. You're utilizing proclamations consistently in case you're aware of it or not. You're demanding and making your work area with each word and thought.

Your feelings are just basic defense models that you heard as a kid. The enormous amounts of those function admirably for you. Various convictions and ideas could likewise be limiting your ability to get the principal assets you say you might want. All that you might want and what you expect your legitimacy could likewise be strange. You do focus on your considerations with the point which it's feasible to begin to wipe out those making encounters you are doing not craving in your life.

If it is anything but an unreasonable measure of issue, seeing every complaint is a certification of something that you figure that you don't require in your life.

At whatever point you isolate; you're guaranteeing that you essentially need more irritation in your life. At whatever point you feel kind of a loss, you're affirming that you need to keep it up, feeling some fortuity. On the off likelihood that you accept that life isn't providing you with what you might want in your reality, in the point, surely, you'll not have the treats which life supplies for others that is before you adjust how you both talk and think.

You do recently never discovered the best approach to talk and talk. People all through the planet are, as of late, beginning to discover our thoughts to make our encounters. Your kin presumably didn't have the haziest idea about it, so they may in no way, shape, or instruct it to you actually. They showed you precisely what things to best like in Life in how their kin advised them. In this way, no one is awesome. Despite the case, it's the correct possibility for us all of us to stir and start to deliberately make our own lives such that suits and reinforces us. You'll, without a doubt, move in the roughage. I will want to move in the grass. We, all in all, may perform it-we ought to decide how. So, what about we set up to accomplish it straightforwardly.

From now into the foreseeable future, I will actually want to talk about certifications as an idea. At that point, I will want to turn out to be excessively explicit about ordinary issues. Likewise, advise you regarding the most awesome approach to carry out positive improvements on your wellbeing, capital, love, life, and so on. This way, you regularly use a little book based on when you're utilized out the structure of assertions, at this stage, you'll utilize the guidelines in many conditions to help you. A couple of people express that "attestations don't work" (that are frequently an insistence in itself) when what they mean is, they don't know how to utilize them accurately. They'll say, "My prosperity is developing," all things considered, at that point, accept, Oh, that is off-kilter, I remember it'll not work. Which insistence does one think will win out? The negative one since it's a cut of a longstanding, proceeding with a point of view on.

A few times, individuals will express their insistences once day by day and issue the rest of the moment. It'll set aside a short effort for assertions to

82

work if they're done that way. The protesting confirmations will consistently win since there is a more prominent volume of those and that they are, for the most part, expressed with phenomenal propensity.

In any circumstance, expressing attestations is basically a tad bit of this cycle.

All that you wrap from the evening and day is essentially huge. The secret to getting your solicitations to work rapidly and steadfastly is to place a climate for them to fill in. Certifications look like seeds planted inland: helpless soil, lacking improvement. Ripe soil, endless event.

The further you choose to think considerations, which empower you to feel better, the faster and better than the insistences work.

Chapter 11 - Psychology for Weight Loss

Weight loss is a long way from being just an actual matter. Numerous significant mental variables lead to stoutness and come in the method of weight loss. To address how weight loss happens mentally, more than truly, we should begin by examining how mental reasons cause stoutness regardless.

Foolish center convictions lead to weight acquires (Annesi et al., 2010).

All that occurs in your life right now is separated through the perspective of these convictions. As far as weight acquire, a few impacts are working in two inverse ways. One works outside-in, which means how you respond to outside occasions by eating, and the other is back to front, which is the component where your psychological framework explores your point of view.

Outside-In Obesity

You are eating more than you need to adapt to various feelings of dread and instabilities. You oppose confronting your feelings of dread and weaknesses as well as your pity and outrage. Since you feel like these sentiments are a lot for you to deal with, your hotel to indulging at whatever point you feel upset. You even hotel to indulging at whatever point you feel exhausted, and at whatever point you feel cheerful because you haven't tracked down the correct approaches to communicate these conclusions. Food utilization is just a route for you to make up for the numerous things that you can't impart in your life. Here are the mental reasons for indulging:

- You are not communicating your requirements.

- You are not communicating your assessments.

- You are smothering your feelings of dread, questions, and frailties.

- The burdens you experience in everyday life get excessively misrepresented in your psyche on account of this.

- Whenever a circumstance or experience triggers your oblivious feelings of trepidation and instabilities, you eat to adapt.

- Your significant negative and nonsensical center convictions never get tended to, and you just keep gaining weight since you deferred defying your weaknesses.

Back to front Obesity

Center convictions control how you see the world, yourself, and others in your life. They are formed since adolescence, from the second you were a defenseless child. You had just two conditions, which are the condition of quiet and the condition of alarm. In the condition of quiet, you were a craze and had a sense of security. In the condition of alarm, you required human contact, food, and consideration. What your requirements were, had incredibly meant for what you look like in the world at this point. To start with, you realized whether the world is a protected spot dependent on whether you were comforted when you were disturbed.

As a little child, parental figures reacted to your requirement for graciousness and love from various perspectives, and not every one of them is correct. How they responded to your displeasure and trouble ingrained numerous oblivious convictions in your psychological framework. Center convictions formed your suspicions on the most fundamental issue, like the accompanying:

- How would others treat you when you need assistance?
- Do you have anybody to depend on?
- Do you have any individual who will hear you out?
- Are you deserving of adoration and consideration?
- What do you have to never really regard and care for?

In a perfect world, a kid will discover that they just need to voice their necessities, and it will be met. Be that as it may, this doesn't occur to everybody. Conventional manners by which youngsters were raised man instructing to forgo communicating rage, and to prevent oneself from crying. Outrage and crying irritated the parental figures. Their primary objective was to stop the articulation as opposed to comforting the kid. How they would do this was by the same token:

- Offering nourishment for the kid to quiet down.
- Avoiding and disregarding the kid, so the youngster understands that crying isn't the best approach to get what they need.
- Punish torment and fierceness as a form of not well-adjusted conduct; These avoidant reactions might have instructed you that there is no reason for opening up. You never figured out how to adapt to your sentiments and correctly express them. You additionally introduced many negative center convictions that unwittingly guided your relationship with food. As you age, you didn't trouble much with good dieting since you didn't see the significance of treating your body with a quality eating routine. You didn't see yourself as adequately significant to contribute. At

87

the point when it came to food and nourishment, you went with the understanding that diet didn't make any difference a lot to your wellbeing. As in all parts of life, the negative center convictions powered low confidence.

In your adolescence and maybe early teenagers, you may have accepted that you are not skillful. Presently, negative center convictions may bring about low confidence. You might be effective outwardly yet have unreasonable assumptions. All the while, negative center convictions reveal to you that you are not fit for meeting these assumptions. In this way, the inward clash is made.

Not exclusively are your suspicions dependent on nonsensical assumptions, yet they are additionally tangled by the negative picture of low self-esteem. It is a heap of harmful sentiments that appears to be practically difficult to escape. Therefore, you eat to recapture, adjust and briefly mitigate the inward struggle.

What care does is that it instructs you to carry these negative convictions to mindfulness and mends them with confidence and sympathy.

For what reason aren't you losing weight?

The explanation that you experience difficulty shedding pounds is that, where it counts, you don't accept that you are skilled or deserving of weight loss. Since what goes within you is so significantly negative and overpowering, you make passionate squares to have the capacity option and adapt to your day-by-day life. The pressure of what goes on inside you just motivations more hunger. Negative self-talk is consistently present although you don't hear the musings deliberately constantly. You might know about the need to get thinner, yet every time you attempt to put forth an attempt, the systems of aversion and self-damage are set off because of a profoundly situated conviction that it is unimaginable for you.

Thus, at whatever point you attempt, you'll experience passionate squares. Enthusiastic squares coming from within are preventing you from adapting to exceptional apprehensions. They cause a bogus hunger. Then again, fears of progress, disappointment, inadequacy, and disgracefulness keep you stuck. This is an endless loop that must be broken with care and self-reflection.

Chapter 12 - Mindset for Weight Loss

Keeping up pounds away is a genuine errand. You would require a solid main impetus for that. After your fruitful excursion of getting in shape, you should search for an explanation sufficiently incredible to encourage you to remain focused. There ought to be a more enthusiastic assent behind each progression that you take, something more powerful than your reasons, something more remunerating than your common routine issues and such. Arriving at your objective weight is without a doubt an accomplishment to celebrate, however fending the pounds off and the fats at the inlet are something to be stressed over as well. No? The rear of your psyche will reply as a YES! In the wake of getting thinner, you will know your body, how it works, the advancement it shows; it's correct, it's horrendous, and everything identified with it. When you complete the excursion of getting more fit effectively, you will have a full comprehension of how your body responds to various sorts of food varieties, every one of the conditions that it manages, and all that it faces.

Here are not many of the focuses which you can remember while battling to avoid the pounds you have once shed:

Quit Restricting Calories

At the point when you limit calories, you put a limit before your body and yourself, and the second you do that; you give a feeling of hardship to your brain because of which it turns out to be more inclined to do over-eating, to enjoy into awful food sources, to leave hands at circumstances where you need to keep a confined bit of food. Try not to check calories. Eat everything with some restraint. Have a reasonable eating routine; there ought to be a decent segment of everything in balance in your dinners. Have partition control. Eat everything except for in little amounts. Try not to indulge and don't gorge. Regardless of whether it is the spotless eating measure or on the off chance that you are taking good suppers, everything ought to be kept to a legitimate extent and ought not to be devoured in bigger amounts.

A decent eating regimen and part control are two of the most fundamental and vital keys to your weight loss upkeep stage. Keep in mind, everything in the limit is the solitary way out.

Stay Active and Stay Accountable

Make yourself cognizant about the way that if you go for awful food decisions and on the off chance that you were over-eat and indulge, you will be rebuffed, and you should be responsible for every one of the insidious and wrong choices. When there is a feeling of responsibility in your sub-cognizant, at that point, you will get cautious before anything that your choice. Therefore, have a diary where you will enter your advance and have a local area or a gathering of individuals who have the very desires as yours, so you are associated with them, you can impart your excursion to them and consequently get the inspiration and that feeling which will help you stay on the track.

Look at Workout as a Lifestyle

Make exercise a lasting piece of your day-by-day schedule. Regardless of whether it is for an hour or the base thirty minutes, do it, and never skip it. Be more grounded than your reasons. Try not to accept it as a discipline and don't think of it as a weight rather, makes it a basic and indivisible piece of your day-by-day schedule, something without which your day will be deficient. Recall that you are your own greatest inspiration. Or then again, all things considered, let me re-state it. You are your ONLY inspiration; therefore, the voice from your inside ought to be adequate to keep you on track and make you traveling as the day progressed. Continue reminding yourself about the easy street that you appreciate after losing all your superfluous fat and weight and thus let your internal identity understand that you are assumed not to kick all your persistent effort into squander, so every effort ought to be added into keeping the weight off. It is your battle, your own special fight, and you are the solitary individual battling it; you are doing it for yourself, for you, your great wellbeing, your own glad and sound life, and your improvement. It includes you and just you; nobody else. Try not to abandon yourself because nobody will come to put resources into you. It is your prosperity and your award, and you should invest heavily in all the difficult work that you do towards it and keep it a steady battle.

Goodbye—Sleep Right

Almost certainly, you won't keep a sound daily schedule and, later, a solid way of life. Give your body adequate rest; it is its fundamental need and prerequisite. Make it vital to set your everyday practice, so that gives you great rest. At the point when you don't rest enough; the odds of reveling in awful food sources are the most extreme since when your body is denied of the measure of rest it ought to be given, it will, in general, feel hungry and pine for awful food varieties and subsequently you may wind up doing pressure eating or enthusiastic eating or reveling into some unacceptable food alternatives. Rest is the essential need of your digestion and your inward frameworks. At the point when they don't get that necessary measure of rest, they won't work accurately, and the odds of your digestion getting slower are at its pinnacle. So recollect that before tallying calories, you need to track the hours of your rest.

Deal with Your Reward System

Recognize your advancement and save a norm of discipline and prize for yourself. We as a whole are people, and people will in general demonstration and live with the idea of discipline and award so when you recognize your triumphs and award yourself with a prize consequently; you will, in general, be more energetic about your objectives and progress, and henceforth you keep on with your excursion much more energetically. The main idea which you need to comprehend after you have shed pounds once. Put forward your week-by-week and month-to-month objectives alive and continue reviving them. Make arrangements and stick to them. Set small targets and attempt to accomplish them. Keep yourself moving. Never skirt an exercise; we never lament any of them. Try not to make colossal arrangements and enormous targets.

Make a Relevant Social Circle

Be a piece of the gatherings that share your desires and objectives. Encircle yourself with positive contemplations and empowering individuals. The main thing which we will, in general, forget while being at a weight-loss venture is that we need a day-by-day portion of inspiration; it is an excursion about self-recuperating, and pessimism is rigorously precluded. In this way, on the off chance that somebody attempts to cut you down, to debilitate you, and to thump you away, simply avoid them. You are now battling so hard with your efforts; don't allow anybody to cut you down.

94

Comprehend your Body

After a long excursion of an effective weight loss measure, you will comprehend your body. You will realize how the frameworks work and how digestion is getting along. Perceive how the body moves and acts as needs to be. Stay away from garbage however much you can. Every one of the fast and prepared food sources is not implied for you; avoid them. The main cause that individuals getting more fit is to avoid low-quality nourishment. Garbage is poison for you, and no one knows it better than you, so don't enjoy it.

Ease Up Sometimes

Permit a cheat supper after like clockwork when you can enjoy your preferred food and not feel awful about it, simultaneously. A cheat supper is fundamental. It permits you to take the food you have been needing. It is required for your extraordinary digestion. It gives a lift to your as of now weight loss in the process excursion, and it will help you not feel denied of the things you needed to enjoy. A cheat feast following a couple of days doesn't make you fat. It will not make you recover every one of the pounds which you have shed as of now. It will keep you fulfilled and fought simultaneously, so don't worry over having a chomp of that pizza you have been obsessed with for some time and don't stress over a cupcake you just ate up, and there is definitely no reason for being stressed over a burger you just had because hello, a solitary dinner will not make you fat and a solitary shake will not allow you to get back every one of the overweight packs you have effectively shed.

Chapter 13 - Why Hypnosis Is the Best Method to Start Weight Loss

Method for weight loss the brain is a mechanism that can keep on changing in the course of our life. The more you listen to this account, the more profound the new propensities and convictions will go.

Realize that it is never too late for positive change. Kindly never listen to this account while driving, working any sort of hardware, while dealing with others, or some other obligations. Kindly make when you can give this 100% your consideration, ideally plunking down in a peaceful space where you won't be intruded. At the point when you're prepared, if it's not too much trouble, get yourself happy with, getting comfortable some time plunking down.

As you sit, simply start to back off. Making time is by all accounts the hardest part, so unwind in realizing that the hardest part is presently finished. As you unwind and get comfortable, simply realize that any development, any change, or anything you need to never really significantly more agreeable, will just guide in your unwinding. Go ahead and move and change on a case-by-case basis.

As you unwind, feeling your body, neck, and head completely upheld, start to interface with your relaxing. Feel your chest rise and fall while easing back down.

Spot all your concentration for the following couple of moments on your breathing, taking in and out gradually. Breathe in quiet and breathing out any musings or pressure and stress, giving up with each breath. Send a flood of unwinding down your whole body and brain. With each breath, let proceed to sink into the floor or seat you are sitting in. Breathing out your negative contemplations, center around sending them away to a better place that you are not centered around.

Follow your breath, realizing that anything huge will return at the correct time. Taking in space into the brain, clearing up adverse musings with each breathe out.

We are relinquishing contemplations, of any strain and additional energy at the top of the priority list.

- I'm easing back down.
- You are tracking down your own speed.

As you breathe, feel your body rise and fall, with the delicate breathe in and breathe out of considerations. Simply believe yourself to give up. With the following breath, center around

sending this breath up and into the face. Feel it liquefying each muscle in the cheeks, up to the eyes, feeling unwinding move through your whole face, releasing and loosening up any strain. Send this as far as possible up into your brow, streamlining any snugness.

With the following breath currently, send it over-top the top of the head, loosening up every one of the muscles encompassing the skull, feeling the rear of your head, and the contact points of the floor or your seat. You were simply feeling your head unwind, sinking back more significantly and more profound. Presently send this breath of unwinding down and around your neck, lengthening and extricating the throat, breathing unreservedly. Open up the aviation routes, and feel every one of the muscles in your neck giving up, unwinding and expanding, feeling it wave to the shoulder bones and down and feeling your shoulder bones sinking further into your seat or your upstanding stance.

Presently send a flood of unwinding to your center, down your stomach, and profound into your hips. Send it down into your seat while sinking. Send the breath down into the fingertips, through the elbows, streaming down into the wrists and hands, topping off totally with quiet and unwinding. Breathe out any resistance, tolerating just peacefully, and send the following breath now down into your legs. Send into your thighs and knees, into your calves, and surprisingly down into your feet to the actual tips of your toes. Give up increasingly more with each breath, dissolving each muscle, and as your breathing gets more familiar and more agreeable as your rest into this space. Envision since your unwinding will develop as I tally you down into more profound levels, starting from 10 to 1.

10. Feel your muscles simply liquefy away, sinking now.

9. Becoming increasingly loose, remaining associated with your breath.

8. Letting go of any last considerations, dissolving them, confiding in this cycle.

7. Coming back to the breath, remaining with the breath.

6. Deep, where it counts.

5. Halfway down now, multiplying your condition of quiet.

4. With your entire body surrendering, permitting gravity to help you from the top of your head to the tips of your toes.

3. Your entire body is getting heavier and heavier; your eyelids are loose.

2. Face loose, jaw loose.

1. Coming to rest, feeling the brain open up in this peaceful place of refuge that is assigned only for you.

As you feel the rest of the world disappear into the foundation, hearing every outer sound and inside sounds mix, as distant sea waves, simply getting more associated with your internal identity, your body sensations, your brain, and feelings. Realize that you are prepared to start your excursion, and realizing that your record is consistently ready, realizing that it will cause you to notice anything pressing in your current circumstance. You can give up, let go totally, and spotlight on the inclination in your body, and the sound of my voice. You realized that all you require to accomplish your objectives exists in you. Notice how you can feel an association in your breath, down into your lungs, getting increasingly more mindful of your psyche and your body.

Notice in what way regularly we are unconscious of the body. We separate the body, from the neck up, and treat nearly everything as an outsider starting from the neck.

Right now is an ideal opportunity to reconnect, to live overall, from the top of your head to the tips of your toes and everything between. Getting mindful of your breathing and your pulse, and expanding on this brain-body association, you are getting increasingly more in-tuned of how shallow or profound your breath is. Of the speed or gradualness of your pulse, and the degree of completion or genuine craving of your stomach. Notice the sentiments in your stomach. Notice the sensitive spots around your mid-region. Would you be able to feel them?

Maybe your stomach mindfulness is simply starting or getting more dependable and will just strengthen. Start to get mindful, feeling your degree of craving or totality, and envision now a size of 1 to 10, or perhaps a dial tone that turns up as you eat. See the numbers plainly marked from 1 to 10, with one being horrendously starving, incapable to consider something besides food, and ten being full, deplorably full, sluggish, and delayed to move.

See the numbers or the scale. Focus on every one of these numbers, and any place you feel this scale, whether around your stomach or to you'd eye, make this as genuine and distinctive as could be expected. Maybe the numbers are red at each finish of the scale when you are starving or excessively stuffed. Between the limits, of 1 starving and ten stuffed, is the sound zone somewhere in the range of 3 and 7 with 3 or 4 where your body calls consideration, with the need to eat: a wonderful vacancy, the expectation of topping off with sustenance, or more noteworthy happiness of food. At the point when you get to the number 7, envision feeling totally satisfied, 3/4 full, still with energy to move, feeling refueled, and prepared to continue ahead with your day, zeroing in on an ideal zone between a three and a 7, never allowing your craving to plunge under a 3, never letting your satisfaction going past a 7 to stuffed.

Similarly that you can and are retraining your mind, with continued listening, you are strengthening your neural organizations, the wiring between your brain and stomach. If whenever you are uncertain, you may stop again for a couple of seconds and serve yourself a cool, reviving glass of water to separate among thirst and certified hunger. If you at any point arrive at a level 3 or on the other hand 4, you will know that the time has come to eat, noticing your ordinary regular cadence of eating, and on the off chance that it is a 5 or above, it is an indication that you need another thing to satisfy you. Maybe actual work to consume off apprehensive strain or possibly a discussion or kind word from a companion. Maybe something to top off your brain, and you will think that it's simpler and

101

more agreeable to distinguish craving from other requirements, other kinds of appetite.

This incorporates enthusiastic craving, mental yearning, or actual appetite, and envisions you presently at home back in the kitchen.

Visualize this scene, notice the shades of the cabinets, the refrigerator, and the broiler.

Feel yourself there, and watch yourself preparing for a feast, requiring a couple of additional seconds before your supper time. Take a couple of full breaths in and out to get quiet and present before each dinner. As you prepare to eat, make the most of your delicate craving. Feel it to gradually fabricate, realizing that with a taste, you will appreciate every significant piece considerably more. Starting with a couple of additional seconds, a couple of moments to put food on a plate or a bowl, and to discover a seat because is putting food on a plate or in a bowl guarantees that it enters your cognizant mindfulness.

Not any more distracted or semi-cognizant eating, full information eating as it were. In the basic demonstration of planning food, giving yourself a spot to sit easily is a demonstration of a sense of pride, regarding yourself as you would a visitor. As you take a gander at the food on a plate or bowl, you'll have a couple of more seconds to take in the smell, the vibe of the supper you are going to appreciate, regarding yourself as perhaps the best visitor.

As you visualize yourself in your kitchen and home, planning food, interfacing with your hunger, diffusing from any feelings identified with your real craving, you understand that you have the right to encounter each significant piece.

That whatever you are placing in your body, you merit the taste, the surface. However much life can be occupied, you transform eating times into needs. Throughout the following not many days, those next couple of moments you provide for the center will venture into minutes, and with each supper, you will back off to a point where you go through at any rate 20 minutes on each dinner. You will start discovering that the mind needs, in any event, 20-minute signs from the stomach, between the second that it is enjoyably satisfied and stimulated. Dial-up, you are inner messages while dialing down on outside messages and distractions. Unwinding and plunking down for each chomp, each supper, each bite.

Chapter 14 - What Is Self-Hypnosis and Its Methods

Self-Hypnosis is perhaps the most impressive thing individuals can accomplish for themselves. It tends to be groundbreaking and change how they identify with themselves and their issues. For a very long time, numerous hypnotists have disagreed with the possibility of self-hypnosis. They accepted that individuals need a mandate voice to control them down the way of their oblivious brain.

Notwithstanding, that is simply false. There are a few different ways you can utilize self-hypnosis to improve your life, make astounding outcomes for yourself, and mend yourself of issues.

From the Swish Pattern to Reframing, they are both incredible assets of self-hypnosis that permit you to change your state, and intensely utilize your hypnosis. You can prepare your mind and build up your points of view.

Self-Hypnosis can be trying to become accustomed to, however, when you understand what you are doing, you can do it rapidly and without any problem.

Record Your Trance

You have figured out how to actuate hypnosis and make a daze. Probably the quickest approaches to make an amazing self-entrancing state are to just record your voice and guide yourself through the interaction with the goal that you can make a powerful, mesmerizing cycle. I realize this may feel like an additional progression to something you will actually want to do without help from anyone else, yet it is fundamental to understand what you can do. Basically, take the recorder from your telephone, record an entrancing meeting, and bring yourself into a daze and utilize that cycle to enter a condition of self-Hypnosis.

Make A Hypnotic Anchor

Before NLP and before hypnosis was utilized all throughout the planet, there was Ivan Pavlov, who was exploring the stomach-related framework through estimations of the salivation in canines. While he was doing this, he saw something bizarre occurring. At last, he saw that the canines appeared to salivate before the food even came. He considered the big picture. In the first place, it was clairvoyant salivation.

Nonetheless, the appropriate response was somewhat more apparent and common, and it was that the ringer that he set up to make sure to take care of the canines on plans had adapted the canines. Each time the chime rang, the canine is relied upon to be taken care of and started to salivate so they could more readily eat the food. The ringing turned into an anchor.

Securing utilizes outer improvements to trigger inner states. It doesn't make any difference what country you need to gather. In case you will feel certain, facilitate your pressure, quit feeling furious, or simply concentrate better. Mooring gives you an incredible asset giving you a stockpile to assume better responsibility for your feelings.

Envision having the option to just and effectively press your fingers together to facilitate a hankering for whatever used to be an obstacle to not acquiescence to. Envision, assuming responsibility for your outrage, and quickly making yourself without a care in the world at a snap of the fingers. Simply envision how stunning and amazing it very well may be to have the option to transform pressure into energy. Envision, taking misery and transform it into imagination. Making anchors can change your daily routine and change how you experience your life. You will be engaged and, above all, be in charge of your life in a way you have never been.

You don't have to have a convoluted or testing life. You have the right to have a phenomenal encounter. Yet, if you don't have authority over your feelings, everything can feel included, and hard. Allow us to get down to how to make a tough anchor for everything without exception you need in your life.

The cycle

Allow us to recall when we tackled visualization and how your brain can't differentiate between an envisioned occasion and the genuine occasion.

That is really critical to understanding all that will occur. This is significant for this interaction. More significant with regards to mooring than envisioning activities, you need to envision feelings. You need to allow your body to feel the inclination you wish to press everything in your body that you would contact when you have that feeling. Whatever feeling you need to feel, regardless of whether it is glad, energized, center, or certain, you realize how these sentiments think, and how your body will feel when you are around there. The more striking you can make that feeling, the better you will be. In this way, let us get to the way toward making a tough anchor that will change your life.

Sort out the Emotion You Want

Glimpse inside yourself and sort out what feeling will serve you. Sort out what feeling will best give you the inspiration and energy you need for whatever state you need to summon.

Envision That Emotion to the Fullest

When you have a reasonable picture of what that feeling is, you need to envision that feeling to the furthest reaches. What's the significance here? It implies you need to understand how that feeling will work out in your body, in your psyche, and in your life. How does your body position itself? Envision every energy without limit.

At the Peak of Emotion, Create an Anchor

At the pinnacle of your passionate state, you need to make the anchor that will actually want to initiate that feeling. You can applaud together, press a few fingers together, step your feet, keep quiet, whatever you need to do, you need to make an actual improvement that you can interface with your enthusiastic state. Each anchor ought to be individualized to the feelings that you need. And you need to ensure that when you make the anchor, you make it at the pinnacle of your enthusiastic strength.

Support It

At the point when you have made the anchor, you need to support it. The way toward fortifying the anchor includes you fractionating from the state and then getting once more into the country. Along these lines, you need to get your psyche out of your enthusiastic state, by adjusting your actual state. Regardless of whether you do some bouncing jacks, or some push-ups, or whatever you need to break the country. At that point, sit down, bring back the feeling, and anchor it once more.

Rehash this cycle a few times, until you begin to feel it, and realize that it is being moored.

Test the Anchor

Whenever you have dealt with each progression, you need to clear your brain again by breaking your state and then testing the anchor to see that it is working. Search for any signs that you are encountering the feelings. Keep in mind, you should do this on numerous occasions to make it perpetual. Yet, on your first time, you ought to have the option to feel some feeling attached to it.

On the off chance that you are working this interaction without anyone else, it will take you additional time, however, you can construct these outcomes. As you do this, you will discover things about your enthusiastic life and your passionate world. As you go through the interaction and make the anchors, you will discover new opportunities and new forces in your passionate control. You will likewise discover how your body makes feelings and how your body structures feelings, giving you a more prominent understanding of your slant. What's the significance here?

After you have made a large group of anchors for enthusiastic states that you need to dominate, presently, the time additionally to make sure to utilize these cycles to make an entrancing state anchor. Regardless of whether you are utilizing the recorded voice method, or one of the systems that I will show you after this, by following a similar technique to make amazing anchors, you can make secures for your entrancing state. This will give you moment admittance to your oblivious brain and the capacity to move your oblivious psyche through self-hypnosis right away. The force of this anchor implies that with a straightforward, loosened-up area, you will actually want to enter a daze voluntarily. This is simply the ideal manner by which to rehearse self-Hypnosis and the quickest path too.

Obviously, the anchor should be developed to do it, and that implies that you should have the option to enter a mesmerizing state to accomplish it.

Obsession, Mantras, and Long Bout Meditation

Self-Hypnosis can be accomplished through a cycle of obsession and mantras.

This may sound new age or religion, yet it is most certainly not. The method of utilizing contemplation to enter a condition of self-hypnosis is very much archived; however, obviously, it is somewhat difficult, as any type of self-hypnosis can be.

Yet, let us give it back. Focus on what`s in from of you, or on the roof on the off chance that you are resting. Relax. Release your body free and let your eyes start to obscure. As you do this, consistent your breathing, and carry your contemplations to your relaxing. In and out, without rushing, every breath profound and filling. As you do this, let your body unwind significantly more.

When you feel totally loose, take a full breath in, and then release it completely, and shut your eyes. Here, you will think about your oblivious, whatever it is, very well may be. For most, it is a room. For a few, it is a cavern. For other people, it is a cave. It doesn't make any difference what it is, yet you will discover what it is to you, and you will enter it. As you open it, you can then walk yourself through the progressions you need. This requires understanding what shifts you need to make and what

110

transforms you need to make before you do it. What illustrations are keeping you down? What splendid future would you like to accomplish?

Everything and anything you would walk somebody through must be now settled and assembled, that you can put it together again in your oblivious.

When it is there, you will test your state, over and again, to ensure that you have it right. You will search for any piece of you that battles against these progressions and address them in your self-actuated state. Every one of these things allows you to make your entrancing state helpful really.

At the point when you initially enter that state, when you feel the total unwinding flush through your body, utilizing secures for that second can be vital and exceptionally accommodating for what's to come. And with that, you have made a self-mesmerizing state.

Self-Hypnosis can be incredible, it very well may be lovely, and it gives you the self-governance to roll out the improvements that you need to make in your life, with or without any other person. It is not troublesome. In any case, it will require some investment. The more you practice, the better you will be eventually.

Chapter 15 - Hypnosis Food Addiction

How to beat food addiction?

Stoutness is a developing scourge on the planet today. It isn't just common among grown-ups, yet the pace of expansion in stoutness among youngsters is significantly stressful. Corpulence has added to the expanded utilization of help, which can uphold weight reduction sponsors like digestion. Food is the endurance capacity of any individual. However, perhaps there is at least one thing like sweets or chocolates that you like more than a few times each day. You may not know; however, these might be pointers of addiction to food. You may likewise be dependent on inexpensive food if you have more cheap food than expected.

The present food addiction resembles a plague. The greatest concern is that numerous individuals who don't realize that they have an infection are still over-alimenting.

The impact is that an individual is dependent on food and burns through a critical number of calories. The clarification that most overweight food customers don't get more fit is because of their dietary patterns.

Doctors recognize these addicts as individuals with voraciously consuming food issues. It can prompt serious issues like diabetes, heart issues, kidney problems, and even melancholy. The critical manifestations of food addiction incorporate a consistent feeling of appetite, moving in mindset, and vacillation in weight.

Treatment and treatment are the best way to deal with the issue of food addiction. You should discover a specialist that can assist you with getting in shape in a facility. On the off chance that you see a specialist, you can realize that you are by all accounts not the only one with this predicament that can assist with lightening the disgrace. An advisor will help you discover why you are dependent and assist you with conquering it with straightforward techniques. He will likewise show you how to shed pounds strongly.

One should likewise perceive that it is a drawn-out measure, so tolerance is fundamental when you meet with a specialist and a clinician, and should submit to their recommendation fittingly and quickly. A few associations run recovery administrations for dietary issues. You can join any of these gatherings too. You need to escape your usual range of familiarity to help yourself manage the addiction and control hunger to dispose of unfortunate foods from your eating regimen.

What foods are destined to be addictive?

The reaction is baffling: commonly, the most scrumptious. A specialist engaged with food reliance assesses the issue in a new report.

His discoveries propose that refined, fat, and high glycemic foods are "all the more regularly associated with food misuse conduct." Here are a few models:

• **Pizza:** Pizza is close to the first spot on the list with its heavenly blend of carbs, salt, and fat. "The number of spikes should I eat?" you at any point pondered. The appropriate response is how to stay away from the pizza call. It ordinarily contains more fat per nibble than other better foods, comprising of many refined fixings. If you join this with salt, you will wind up with an extraordinary formula to get dopamine directly to the following tip. You realize it's not fundamental, but rather than your brain advises you.

- **Treats:** Sugar and fat will rapidly instigate the brain to want more, sweets, treats, cake, and frozen yogurt. A pungent dinner is a normal practice with a sweet pastry, yet it's anything but a protected alternative. It permits you to devour sugar and burn through an overabundance if your food alternative is undesirable. In this manner, you can have the additional advantage of calories, fat, and sugar.
- **Seared foods:** This model isn't amazing thinking about what we definitely know. Freezes and potato chips are salted and normally cooked in oils that don't do your body or mind a lot of good.

Albeit some seared foods are delightful, they are undesirable and defenseless against food addiction.

Shouldn't something be said about carbonated beverages?

Sodas and greasy and pungent foods can be addictive. An examination completed in 2007 tracked down a protected association between the utilization of carbonated foods and expanded energy admission, that is, the utilization of more calories daily, notwithstanding the current relationship among them and the antagonistic impacts on diet and wellbeing just as weight acquire. Carbonated drinks were regularly connected with a diminished utilization of calcium and different supplements.

Buyers of soda pops are considerably more in danger for long-haul clinical issues.

How do carbonated beverages turn out to be so addictive? The secret is clear to open up: normal carbonated beverages are loaded up with sugar and regularly additionally with caffeine.

Studies show that such drinks can assist with weight acquire because counterfeit sugars are designed to cause comparable responses in the mind.

One exploration expressly demonstrates that people who devour counterfeit sugars as of now may have an expanded craving for sugar, pick sugar over better foods, and be less persuaded by wellbeing.

Steps to Control Food Addiction

1. Distinguish the foods you are dependent on

The most addictive foods are wealthy in sugars, fat, flour, and sodium. Also charged foods like espresso, sodas, and chocolate.

2. Make a solid substitution

At the point when the inclination to fulfill your addiction hits, eat another better food. At the point when sugar levels drop, hunger hits. Rather than burning through sugar, eat solid protein every 3 or 4 hours, for example, cashew or Pará nuts. Wipeout soda pops (even dietary ones) and industrialized juices (which have a high convergence of sugar). Take unsweetened water and regular squeezes, all things considered. A few fluids, similar to squeezed orange, are extremely caloric. Really like to eat the natural product with bagasse.

Remember breakfast. It is the main dinner of the day. It should contain organic products, oats, and protein. At the point when we don't have breakfast, the longing to eat the food we are dependent on can be wild.

3. Drink, rather than eating

A glass of water might be the answer for what you believe is hunger, yet which is thirst.

4. Involve your time and your brain

Abstain from doing nothing when you are not working or contemplating. The more things you need to do, the less time you'll need to consider food.

5. Practice actual activities

Eating something we like a great deal creates a feeling of delight. Actual activities likewise incite such sentiments. The thing that matters is that after active work, you will feel fulfilled and be feeling acceptable, while when you gorge, you will feel pitiful and regretful. Practicing supports confidence, and gorging at last influences confidence.

6. Purchase quality foods

When shopping at the grocery store, try not to go through the sweet's paths, particularly if your object of condemnation is around there. Make a rundown of incredible items for your wellbeing and follow them when shopping.

7. Learn or relearn how to bite

Bite gradually and altogether. Legitimate biting produces satiety and great processing. The stomach sends a satiety message to the mind following a little way from the beginning of the dinner. The more you bite, the more it will take to eat.

You will be satiated with significantly short of what you think. Hence, it is fundamental that you permit around 30 minutes to eat your primary dinners.

8.   Look for master exhortation

Pigging out is an illness, so it should be suitably treated. Without the help of a clinician, nutritionist, and differently trained professionals, you will think that it's difficult to do the treatment until the end. Backslides can be progressive, which can be a justification for debilitation and withdrawal.

Beat Your Food Addiction and Lose Weight!

At the point when you hear "addiction," you, for the most part, consider narcotics or smoking addiction. They stop nearly nothing and consider turning out to be food-dependent. You can get dependent as fast as you can with prescriptions. Despondency has a critical impact, yet there are numerous clarifications regarding why it is conceivable.

A portion of the appropriate responses is that you are exhausted and need to have some food or mental issues you don't think about. How might you respond if you realize you are food-enduring at this point?

You should initially take a full breath and know it's alright. Try not to let frenzy and uneasiness prevent you from making the best decision in your way. Inhale out at this point.

You might need to do it several seconds before you feel loose. You need to zero in on intuition decidedly before you intend to accomplish something and understand that you can vanquish this addiction. The second you keep on living contrarily with food is the point at which you are dependent. Know, "I shed pounds, and I'm protected." Don't consider saying, "I ought to get in shape," regardless of whether it's in the present and "now" tense, and you make it future tense. Since you are correct, the following move ought not to be such a test.

Discover a specialist who can assist you with succeeding in a weight-reduction plan. Joining a program helps you since you're cognizant that you're in good company, and you can discover a few times what made you dependent on food in any case.

You will be shown a better method to shed pounds and vanquish your addiction by going to a center. From the outset, it probably won't be helpful, however at long last, it is very granting.

You should toss out the entirety of your inexpensive food while you're doing the arrangement. This will be a critical change for some. Tossing out some unacceptable food will assemble a surprisingly better mentality since you realize that you can do it without a doubt.

Chapter 16 - Deep Sleep Meditation and Rapid Weight Loss

Nowadays, weight loss remains a very popular topic. There are many ways to lose weight, but in today's day and age, where time is of the essence, rapid weight loss methods might be just what you need. Here, we will go over three effective and well-known methods for aiding your diet and your busy lifestyle:

Rapid Weight Loss Hypnosis and Deep Sleep Meditation

Rapid Weight Loss Hypnosis and Deep Sleep Meditation are two methods of reducing the stress that can help improve your mood as well as combat potential cravings for sweets or other foods high in calories. Generally, people who practice meditation are shown to be able to reduce their weight. They also have a better focus on their diet and feel better about themselves. You may be surprised as to just how effective this simple exercise can be in helping you reduce stress and achieve your weight loss goals.

Hypnosis is one of the most effective methods of therapy for deep relaxation and enhancing personal growth. It is a mental means by which an individual can achieve deep and therapeutic relaxation through self-suggestion during hypnosis sessions. If you are looking for deeper levels of sleep, hypnosis can help you get there...

First up, we have Rapid Weight Loss Hypnosis. [**NOTE:** the following information is for informational purposes only and should not be considered medical advice. If you are experiencing weight loss-related health issues, it is recommended that you speak with your physician or an alternative health care provider.]

What is Rapid Weight Loss Hypnosis?

Rapid Weight Loss Hypnosis uses a combination of hypnosis and positive affirmations to help induce a deep state of hypnagogic trance (a trance-like state that precedes sleep) and activate the subconscious mind. Through chanting affirmations, such as "I am healthy, fit, and strong," repetitively while in this trance-like state, the subconscious mind accepts these "new truths" as facts.

What are some of the benefits of Rapid Weight Loss Hypnosis? Rapid Weight Loss Hypnosis is effective in reducing stress and improving mood. This process enables the body to respond more quickly to suggestions or commands, thereby helping to achieve your weight loss goal faster and with greater success.

How does Rapid Weight Loss Hypnosis work?

Rapid Weight Loss Hypnosis uses an intense relaxation response. It also involves a focus on positive affirmations and self-hypnosis, which increase confidence, improve self-esteem and give you a sense of well-being as you move toward your goals.

What is Deep Sleep Meditation?

Deep Sleep Meditation is an advanced practice of meditation that can help you achieve deep and restful sleep at night. Deep Sleep Meditation involves a deep state of relaxation during sleep as one sleeps in a comfortable position. This type of meditation helps reduce stress and promotes a sense of calmness, helping you to relax before you sleep.

What are some of the benefits of Deep Sleep Meditation?

Deep Sleep Meditation is very effective in achieving deep and restful sleep, which can help you relax and feel well-rested the next day. Deep Sleep Meditation is also known to help increase alertness and improve concentration during the day, leading to better academic performance at school or work.

Is there anything else I should know about Rapid Weight Loss Hypnosis? There are many ways to achieve your weight loss goals. The more you know, the better you will be able to help yourself. Rapid Weight Loss Hypnosis can also help you learn how to change your eating habits and learn how to cope with stress through several steps, as well as giving you the tools and knowledge that will give you success in achieving your weight loss goals.

Chapter 17 - Healthy Food Hypnosis

You as of now, comprehend the significance of sustenance and why you need to figure out how to advance it. Be that as it may, the subsequent inquiry is, how regularly would it be advisable for you to eat? Numerous individuals don't pose themselves this inquiry since they eat when they're ravenous. Odds would you say you are, do the equivalent because, after all the body shouts, it's eager when it's searching for additional supplements, correct? Indeed, that is in part obvious. For example, think about the time, you out of nowhere, get a hankering for red meat or spinach. That is frequently a sign that you need iron, and your body is searching for foods that are wealthy in that specific supplement.

Notwithstanding, your body is additionally impacted by your craving to encounter joy, joy, and unwinding. Food does that to you. It eases your nervousness, it gives you a snapshot of euphoria, and it by and large loosens up you.

On account of the issues referenced above, we need rules. We need data so we can settle on the correct decision and not simply indiscriminately follow our desires. Our minds get joy from fats and sugars on account of an antiquated sense to fill out for our endurance, in addition to other things. Nonetheless, we can't permit ourselves to follow this nature any longer. This is one reason why a few exploration establishments thought of five times a day feast plan. The new arrangement was intended to show individuals eating vegetables and organic products all the more frequently. At times, it was encouraged to have up to nine suppers per day, generally comprising of foods grown from the ground. Yet, let's be honest, who has the opportunity to every, substantially less get ready or cook five to nine little dinners day by day?

Eating frequently, particularly products of the soil, has improved the general wellbeing insights. The training endeavors of governments have driven individuals to burn through much less immersed fat and eat more leafy foods. This by itself has shown that practicing good eating habits isn't just about the number of calories you burn through. It's fundamental to get the correct sort of supplements. It's not the equivalent for your heart and veins on the off chance that you eat an apple, or it is identical in potato chips that are absorbed immersed fats.

Brief Guide to a Healthy Diet

Eating the correct things is fundamental, however, this isn't THE answer for the entirety of our medical conditions brought about by our dietary patterns. To live soundly, we need to utilize various instruments. To stay with our vehicle similarity from prior, it's insufficient to continue to feel the vehicle with gas, we likewise need to deal with it by replacing its oil, and ensuring everything is as indicated by specs. Our bodies work the same way. Thus, one of the primary things we need to figure out is keeping a healthy load through wellness.

We as a whole know at this point that being overweight isn't healthy. Regardless of what drives an individual to be large, that isn't useful for the heart, and the person can create diabetes and other medical problems. Furthermore, if you are overweight, you should join a healthy eating plan with a lot of actual work. This can be an issue for some these days. Simply think about all the workplace occupations out there. You may be working in an office yourself. What does your day resemble? On the off chance that you get up, shower, eat, drive to work, go through 9 hours at a work area, drive back home, watch Netflix, rest, and rehash, at that point, chances are your body isn't fit. Simply remember that you can likewise be thin or at normal body weight, yet that doesn't mean you're healthy. An excessive number of individuals believe they're excellent because they aren't overweight.

Practicing is significant. Wellness is to sustenance what Yin is to Yang. We need active work to keep the heart healthy, to keep up bulk, and to get a portion of energy. Not practicing can cause us generally to feel drained and lazy. Nonetheless, we can rapidly fix this!

You should simply add a 30 min time of actual work each day. Assuming you are chiefly stationary, you can begin with even less movement and steadily increment it. This isn't pretty much as alarming as it sounds, regardless. You don't really need to get running at 6 AM, and you don't have to pay for rec center participation by the same token. You should simply roll out little improvements consistently. For example, you can stroll to the workplace if you don't live the greater part an hour away. You can likewise dump the vehicle for a bike.

You'd be astounded how much distance you can cover on a bicycle, and it's a lot more affordable. Consume calories and fat rather than gas. It's appropriate for you, and nature too, which is a reward.

On the off chance that strolling or cycling is not feasible, you can do various activities at home, or even at the workplace, with only your body weight. Look at certain recordings on home wellness on YouTube.

When you have your wellness routine under control, you need to investigate your decision in food. Here you can utilize the food pyramid as a guide, and pick a wide assortment of nutritious foods.

Did you realize that your body needs, in any event, around 40 supplements to work at an ideal level? It seems as though a great deal, however, if you keep your eating regimen changed, you can acquire every one of them. Additionally, a fluctuated diet will likewise hold you back from getting exhausted. We normally partner eats fewer carbs, and "healthy" with exhausting. In any case, that is a result of terrible publicizing and your folks shouting at you to eat all your food, regardless of whether you didn't care for it (my foe was broccoli). It doesn't need to be that way, not today, with such countless methods of cooking each conceivable fixing. Simply consider the number of societies there are on Earth, and everyone has built up an alternate method of cooking things like broccoli. Energizing!

To rapidly oversee your eating regimen, you should begin by choosing a wide assortment of entire grains. Grains are plentiful in fiber, minerals, nutrients, and different other natural mixtures that are essential for limiting the danger of coronary illness and different issues that show up with age. Then, you need foods grown from the ground. They are wealthy in supplements and don't have any fat. Simply ensure you eat them as opposed to drinking them. That squeezed orange may be delectable, yet you're leaving behind most supplements that are found in the mash and internal linings of the organic product. At the point when you drink a couple of oranges, for example, rather than eating one, you may, in any case, get a few supplements, yet you are devouring, for the most part, sugars and void calories. Along these lines, eat your leafy foods, or "drink" them entire, not simply crushed.

At long last, you need to settle on the correct decisions similarly as with anything throughout everyday life. You need to begin giving close consideration to the wholesome substance mark on the pack of whatever you purchase. If you need to become familiar with the dietary benefit of different natural products, since they don't accompany a name normally, you are a Google search away from the appropriate response. Just sort something like "healthy benefit of an orange." Other than that, you can adhere to things you presumably definitely know, similar to fats, sugars, salt, and liquor being typically awful for you if not burned through sparingly.

We looked at what practicing good eating habits means and why we need to focus on sustenance as a rule. Before you begin rolling out huge improvements to your life and your eating regimen, you need to make a stride back and investigate where you are at this moment. Be straightforward with yourself and recognize the issues so you can address them each in turn. Simply remember that nourishment is a part of your whole way of life. At the point when you work on rolling out healthy improvements to get the appropriate sustenance, your body, and your brain need, you are making a drawn-out responsibility. Thus, take as much time as is needed to shape a relationship with yourself and the food you eat. Eat strongly, rest better.

Studies have insisted that distinctive sustenance stuff (lettuce, nuts, kiwis, natural products, and altogether more) increases rest length and rest quality. A continuous report from experts at the University of Extremadura certified this for organic products, for instance. These experts found that melatonin levels in their exploratory gatherings extended by and large.

It has been found that tart organic products (the unforgiving kind) are a trademark wellspring of melatonin. In this manner, drinking cherry crush or having it like it before bed may improve your rest quality. There are even some little examinations like those drove at the University of Rochester Medical Center in New York, and the School of Life Sciences at Northumbria University in the UK have proposed uniting tart natural products into your step by step diet to help direct your rest cycle and simplify it for you to fall asleep around evening time.

Moreover, lettuce is a stunning, convincing rest time partition that helps with rest. So, if you're feeling puckish after the sun goes down, chow down on a part of that firm green stuff and like some shut-eye.

Chapter 18 - Daily Motivation with Mini Habits

Affirmations are an incredible tool to use close by hypnosis to assist you with overhauling your mind and improve your weight reduction capacities. Certifications are fundamentally an instrument that you use to help you to remember your picked "revamping" and to urge your psyche to select your more current, better mentality over your old unfortunate one. Utilizing Affirmations is a fundamental piece of mooring your hypnosis endeavors into your day-by-day life, so, basically, you use them on a standard premise.

When utilizing affirmations, it is fundamental that you use those that are significant and that will uphold you in securing your picked reality into your current reality. We will investigate absolutely what Affirmations are and how they work, how to pick ones that will function for you, and 300

Insistences that will help set you on your way.

What Are Affirmations, and How Do They Work?

Whenever you rehash something to yourself so anyone can hear, or in your musings, you are certifying something to yourself. We use affirmations reliably if we deliberately acknowledge them. For instance, if you are on your weight reduction excursion and you rehash "I'm never going to lose the weight" to yourself routinely, you are attesting to yourself that you are never going to prevail with weight reduction. Moreover, if you are reliably saying, "I will consistently be fat" or "I'm never going to arrive at my objectives," you are certifying those things to yourself, as well.

At the point when we use affirmations unexpectedly, we regularly end up utilizing affirmations that can be frightful and hurtful to our minds and our world.

You may wind up securing in turning into a psychological harasser toward yourself as you reliably rehash things to yourself that are harsh and surprisingly absolutely mean. As you do this, you certify a lower ability to be self-aware certainty, an absence of motivation, and a guarantee to a body shape and wellbeing venture that you would prefer not to keep up.

Attestations, regardless of whether positive or negative, cognizant, or oblivious, are continually making or building up the capacity of your brain and mentality. Each time you rehash something to yourself, your psyche mind hears it and endeavors to make it a piece of your existence. This is because your psyche mind is liable for making your reality and your feeling of character. It builds up both around your affirmations since these are what you see, similar to your unadulterated fact of the matter; in this manner, they make a "solid" establishment for your world and personality to lay on. On the off chance that you need to change these two parts of yourself and your experience, you will have to change what you are regularly rehashing to yourself, so you are done making a reality and character established in pessimism.

To change your psyche experience, you need to deliberately pick positive affirmations and rehash them generally to assist you with accomplishing the truth and character that you really need. Along these lines, you are bound to make an encounter that reflects what you are searching for, as opposed to an encounter that reflects what your cognizant and subliminal brain has consequently gotten on.

How Do I Pick and Use Affirmations for Weight Loss?

Picking Affirmations for your weight reduction venture requires you first to comprehend what it is that you are searching for, and what kinds of positive contemplations will assist you with getting. You can begin by distinguishing what your fantasy is, the thing that you need your optimal body to closely resemble, and how you need to feel as you accomplish your considered getting in shape. Whenever you have distinguished what your vision is, you need to figure out what current convictions you have around the fantasy that you are seeking to accomplish. For instance, if you need to shed 25 pounds so you can have better weight, however, you accept that it will be inconceivably difficult to lose that weight, at that point, you realize that your present convictions are that getting thinner is difficult. You need to distinguish every agreement encompassing your weight reduction objectives and perceive which ones are negative or are restricting and keeping you from accomplishing your objective of getting in shape.

After you have distinguished which of your convictions are negative and pointless, you can pick Affirmations that will help you change your convictions.

Commonly, you need to choose an assertion that will assist you with changing that faith the other way. For instance, on the off chance that you think "getting thinner is hard," your new confirmation could be "I lose the weight easily." Even if you don't accept this further assertion at present, the objective is to rehash it to yourself enough that it turns into a piece of your character and, definitely, your existence. Along these lines, you are mooring in your

Entrancing meetings and you are successfully revamping your brain in the middle of meetings, as well.

133

As you use Affirmations to assist you with accomplishing weight reduction, I urge you to do such in a manner that is natural to your experience. There is no set-in-stone manner to move toward affirmations, as long as you are utilizing them consistently. When you feel yourself easily having confidence in confirmation, you can begin consolidating new affirmations into your routine so you can keep on utilizing your affirmations to improve your prosperity in general. In a perfect world, you ought to consistently be utilizing positive Affirmations even after you have seen the progressions you want, as affirmations are an incredible method to help normally keep up your psychological, enthusiastic, and actual prosperity.

How Are Affirmations Going to Help Me Lose Weight?

Confirmations will assist you with shedding pounds in a couple of various ways. Above all else, and likely generally self-evident is the way that Affirmations will assist you with getting the outlook of weight reduction. To lay it out plainly: you can't lounge around accepting nothing will work and anticipate that things should work for you. You should have the option to develop a propelled attitude that permits you to make achievements. If you can't really accept that it will work out as expected: believe that it won't materialize.

As your mentality improves, your psyche mind will begin changing different things within your body, as well. For instance, instead of making wants and desires for things that are not beneficial for you, your body will start to make needs and requirements for things that are sound for you. It will likewise quit making internal clashes around settling on the correct decisions and dealing with yourself. You may even end up experiencing passionate feelings for your new eating regimen and your new exercise schedule. You will likewise likely end up normally inclining toward practices and habits that are better for you without making a decent attempt to make those habits. As a rule, you may create habits that are sound for you without understanding that you are making those habits.

Maybe than having to intentionally get mindful of the requirement for addictions, and afterward placing in the work to create them, your body and psyche will normally start to perceive the requirement for better pursues and will make those routines for the most part too.

A few investigations have likewise proposed that utilizing affirmations will help your brain and subliminal brain unexpectedly administer your body, as well. For instance, you might have the option to improve your body's capacity to process things and deal with your weight normally by utilizing affirmations and hypnosis. In doing as such, you might have the option to subliminally change which chemicals, synthetic substances, and catalysts are made within your body to assist with things like stomach-related capacities, energy creation, and other weight-and well-being related worries that you may have.

Certifications for Healthier Habits

Your habits can assume a critical part of your health. From how you eat to how you rest and how you, in any case, deal with yourself, rehearses are fundamental. As you run after getting thinner and making a better way of life, positive affirmations can help you. With the accompanying positive Affirmations, you can make focusing on your better habits substantially more direct.

- It is simple for me to have better habits.
- I make some simple memories of eating good food.

- I eat consistently.

- I decide to eat good food sources.

- I move my body consistently.

- I encourage sound habits, so I can appreciate a solid body.

- I generally pick the solid choice.

- I deal with my body in the most ideal manner conceivable.

- I'm committed to dealing with my body.

- Solid habits fall into place easily for me.

- I'm centered around carrying on with a better life.

- I'm turning into a better individual every day.

- I'm figuring out how to settle on better decisions.

- I decide to eat just quality food varieties.

- I'm getting better on account of my solid habits.

- I take the best consideration of my body.

- Solid habits are simple habits.

- I'm becoming familiar with better habits every day.

- I rest when my body needs rest.

- I practice when my body needs to move.

- I give my body precisely what it needs to remain sound.

- I'm continually figuring out how to have better habits.

- I deal with my body with solid schedules.

- Solid schedules make it simple for me to deal with my body.

- I make sound habits and schedules that serve my interesting necessities.

- I deal with my body the way my body needs me to.

- I'm willing to figure out how to deal with my interesting body.

- I generally put exertion into understanding my body's necessities.

- I instruct myself on solid habits and authorize them however much I can.

- I'm improving at keeping up my solid habits every day.

- I fuel my body with solid habits.

- I love participating in solid habits that cause me to feel better.

- My body feels great when I carry on with a solid life.

- Solid habits fulfill me.

- I encourage better habits in all aspects of my life.

- I revere having a better whole self.

- I live to make the best consideration of myself and my body.

- I make some simple memories encouraging new habits.

- My old habits shed with ease.

- I make ready for better habits to exist in my life.

Chapter 19 - Power of Guided Meditation

A quarter of a year later, Bonnie weighed 62 kilos (137 lbs.), and she felt lovely. She felt lovely and not just from her viewpoint. Additionally, the rest of the world saw her as delightful. She spread certainty, energy, and internal harmony. She wasn't thin yet, yet she was fit as a fiddle. It wasn't hard to track down a person who appreciated the new Bonnie. Interestingly, she became hopelessly enamored and experienced genuine joy. She met Tony in a treatment bunch where the members were sharing their self-assessment issues. The two of them had been going to the gathering for a year. Bonnie saw Tony very quickly; however, it wasn't corresponding initially. As Bonnie was getting thinner, she was getting more 'apparent' to Tony. Bonnie knew about the explanation Tony began to show interest toward her was a result of her appearance. Be that as it may, she needed to neglect this to have the option to live her first kiss, embrace, and appreciate heartfelt suppers. She started to see the value in her appearance, and she intended to turn it out to be more excellent. Why? Since her psyche associated her thriving romantic tale with her unfathomable look.

Likewise, she went on her eating routine program since she would not like to stop at 62 kilos (137 lbs.). Past self-hypnosis, she took in its related strategy: meditation. I'll disclose to you why she has discovered meditation so dynamic for weight reduction.

What is meditation?

Meditation comes from "medication," which is a Latin word and initially implies normal medication. Meditation implies that we don't distinguish our contemplations with the voice and feelings in our minds, yet go past them and notice them impartially without negative or good decisions. This method can be polished even while cleaning, and we needn't bother with explicit conditions to contemplate. If we accomplish something from the heart, we can say that we are considering. Meditation is the craft of altogether diverting concentration to only a certain something.

Meditation is a changed condition of mindfulness that can't be delivered by will or constrained. In such a manner, it is like rest, because the more we need to rest, the more ready we will be. Meditation, for the most part, alludes to a perspective whereby the body is intentionally cheerful and loose, and our soul has relinquished harmony and focus inside ourselves. Meditation doesn't only suggest sitting or resting for 5 to 10 minutes peacefully. Meditation in reality requests careful work. The brain should be loose and adjusted. Simultaneously, the mind should be ready with the goal that it doesn't permit any upsetting contemplations or wants to infiltrate. We start meditation with our work. All things considered, when we dig seriously into ourselves, we see that it isn't ourselves that permits us to enter the condition of meditation. The Supreme or Creator contemplates inside and through us, with our purposeful consideration and authorization.

The point is to look for harmony and independence from upsetting contemplations. In such cases, the meditator accomplishes a break from the climate so that from a mental perspective, the experience could even be known as a changed condition of cognizance. At the point when we can make our psyches quiet and still, we will contact another presence stirred inside us. On the off chance that our brain is released and serene, and our general existence turns into an unfilled vessel, at that point, our inner presence can call upon unceasing harmony, light, and benevolence to stream into and fill this vessel. This occurs during meditation.

The impact of meditation

Meditation has been utilized in numerous societies for millennia on account of its various advantages: it diminishes nervousness and causes individuals to feel glad. Temporarily, meditation enjoys mostly mental benefits, yet over the long haul, it has actual results. The individuals who attempt meditation can make the most of its advantages in the present moment like equilibrium, more prominent harmony and imperativeness, and a diminished requirement for rest. Actual impacts can be knowledgeable about only a couple of months: in addition to other things, a pulse may get back to business as usual, or processing may improve. So you can envision how gainful it very well may be over the long haul.

The University of California's Neuroscience Laboratory has been investigating the effects of meditation on the brain's construction for quite a long time. Their latest exploration has concentrated long-haul impacts in the personalities of standard meditators contrasted with non-meditators. As per their outcomes, the cerebral cortex of long haul meditators is more set apart than that of non-meditators, demonstrating expanded intellectual execution. The Frontiers in Human Neuroscience distributed exploration, which turned into achievement in science since it has for some time been accepted that the mind mass arrives at its top in the mid-twenties and afterward starts to limit gradually (Bae, Hur, Hwang, Jung, Kang, Kim, Kwak, Kwon, Lee, Lim, Cho, and Park, 2019). it was an inescapable assessment that there was no real way to intrude on this cycle. In any case, it is currently realized that the mind holds its versatility somewhat, and it can actually change because of meditation. Prior investigations have shown that for long-term meditators, both dark matter and white matter in the mind have expanded in weight. (The previous contains the cells of the mental nerve cells; the last incorporates the neuronal cell-shaping projections). The number of neurons in the cortex changes without a doubt, seldom in adulthood. One gathering of the momentum research included 28 men and 22 ladies, their normal age was 51, and they had all been pondering for a normal of 20 years. The most established member was 71, and the most experienced meditator had been rehearsing day by day for a very long time.

The specialists performed MRI sweeps of members' minds and contrasted them with 50 non-thinking individuals from the benchmark group.

Ordinary practice can build the benefits of meditation. As per research, the more professionals rehashed profound breathing strategies and other meditation techniques, the more they alleviated the manifestations of joint inflammation, diminished their agony, expanded their insusceptible frameworks, showed better chemical levels, and brought down pulse. As per the scientists, this clarifies that an individual's psychological state can change his state of being and gives an additional inspiration to why conventional Tibetan, Indian, and Ayurvedic medication see meditation and the redundancy of mantras as restorative.

Many logical records affirm the positive mending and medical advantages of meditation. Here are some of them.

During the initial 20 minutes of meditation, digestion is decreased by sixteen percent. The body profoundly quiets down during supernatural meditation, which is the consequence of diminished cell oxygen use because of decreased digestion. It likewise diminishes pulse and balances out blood dissemination (Dillbeck and Orne-Johnson, 1987). In addition, the pulse drops, and solid pressure and uneasiness thusly vanish. Meditation has been demonstrated to be compelling in defeating persistent dread and expanding confidence (Eppley, Abrams, and Shear, 1989). Meditation is additionally a viable method to make unwinding and diminish physiological incitement. The pith of the marvel is a lessening in respiratory rate, oxygen utilization, and carbon dioxide exhalation. Breathing isn't just more extraordinary however, more profound, imperative limit increments from resting 450-550 ml to 800-1300 ml (up to 2000 ml for some expert meditators) and stays steady all through. In any case, a lower respiratory rate isn't offset by more profound breathing, coming about in a 20% decrease in respiratory volume under rest.

A few games clinicians feel that meditation might be fitting for improving athletic execution (Syer, and Conolly, 1984). Meditation can help decrease the pressure of rivalry; however, with some training, a competitor can likewise figure out how to loosen up various muscle bunches separately and distinguish complex contrasts in muscle strain.

All through meditation, the competitor can expect the following occasion (like skiing downhill) in such detail that the representation of the activity can be, for the most part, synchronized with the actual development. The skier expects how he will begin from the beginning position, floating down and speeding up, staying away from the entryways, and doing the whole race in his mind. By outlining pictures of fruitful execution, a competitor may endeavor to program their muscles and body for the best outcomes.

The power of meditation

Meditation has great power since we partner feelings coming from the profundities of the spirit with cognizant ideas. In meditation, the individual is brought into a similar recurrence as the beginning of the Inner Self, that is, the actual Universe, and in this manner is straightforwardly associated with the cognizance circle of the Universe. In this state, there is no time limit, so the pictured satisfaction can promptly extend to the actual level. Because of customary meditation, we get various advantages in a physical and mental sense. We will be better because when we center around our breathing, our circulatory strain drops, and our pulse eases back down; therefore, we become more settled. It assists us with having a more clear psyche, figure out our considerations and feelings, making our correspondence more profitable both at work and in public activity.

We can concentrate all the more effectively and appropriately feel less focused. We become more mindful of our feelings; subsequently, we can oversee them all the more adequately.

We discover an answer sooner in parts of our lives where we feel stuck. It advances the handling of mental issues. It assists with discovering harmony and equilibrium. We draw nearer to getting ourselves, individuals around us, our lives, and our central goal. At the point when we acknowledge ourselves as we will be, we got positive, upbeat, and alluring. This will make our current relationship more personal or, if we are separated from everyone else, the ideal accomplice will come into our lives.

Chapter 20 - How to Practice Every Day

For your fast exercise schedule, stroll up through the steps at the office. Park your vehicle at the farthest spot and trip as far as possible distance. Take your canine on a long walk. Take part all around you can. That is the objective of working out. If you miss any exercise or you were unable to get rolling one day, don't simply hang up on it, and simply refocus the following day.

Set a daily schedule for regular Hypnosis meditation and certification for weight reduction

On the off chance that you are stuck in the normal, worn-out heart stimulating exercise classes, you could blend things up and attempt to take another class at your rec center. The absolute most blazing rec center classes that you could be thinking about incorporate indoor cycling, boxing-based projects, yoga classes, trapeze artistry, and military workmanship. This can assist you with combating fatigue, which is the main motivation behind why you partake in enthusiastic eating and quit working out. Attempt consistently to drink a lot of water while utilizing it. Warm-up before working out. On the off chance that you haven't heated up, you need to start heating up before each activity. Make it a propensity to heat up. It isn't important to heat up before any exhausting activity, yet thusly, you'll have the option to get your blood streaming, and you have the option to set yourself up for any action ahead.

Standing Reach Stretch

One of the extending practices that you can do is the standing arrive at a stretch. This stretch includes the chest area's development. Along these lines, start with your arms, hold your arms straight down, other than your body's with your palms confronting in reverse. Utilize one arm, raise it forward, and fabricate it as high as could really be expected.

Presently fix your abs and utilize the contrary arm to contact your shoulders and stretch across your chest somewhat. Presently hold the stretch for 10 to 30 seconds. Rehash a similar stretch with your arms coming the other way.

The neck extends the chest and backstretch. Utilize your hands to get the closures of a little towel on the two sides. Presently carry your arms to the chest level and somewhat fold on the footing of the sheet and hold it for around 10 to 30 seconds.

Neck Stretch

The neck stretch is the chest area stretch. This stretch is ideal for golf players.

Get the finish of a little towel with your decision, and marginally fold them to the finish of the divider.

The chest and Shoulders stretch

Presently the following stretch is the chest and shoulder stretch. This stretch is fantastic in the wake of swimming. So take your hands behind you, and hold the finish of a towel at your hip. Presently raise your chest high and raise your arms forward now, hold the stretch for around 30 seconds.

Quadriceps Stretch

The following stretch is the quadriceps stretch. This stretch is appropriate for sprinters, high-cut cyclists, and walkers. Sit behind the seat and clutch the seat for equilibrium and backing. Presently take one hand and get your other lower leg. Tenderly push your foot forward towards your overabundances. Try not to fold or lean forward however, keep your chest lifted high. Presently do this stretch for around 10 to 30 seconds.

Presently rehash exactly the same thing utilizing the other leg.

Standing external thigh stretch

Remain behind the seat, and clutch the rear of the seat for balance. Spot one of your feet behind the seat and askew press your impact points to the floor.

Hold the stretch for around 30 seconds and put it doing utilizing your other leg.

Ligament Stretch Arm's Length

The following stretch is the ligament stretch stand. Keep your a safe distance behind the seat and clutch the rear of the seat to help and adjust yourself.

Presently keep your feet a couple of inches from your toes why you guide your impact points toward the ground. Gradually push your pelvis while twisting your elbows and inclining forward. Backing yourself with your hands to the rear of the seat.

Presently do this for around 30 seconds.

Standing slim stretch stand

The following stretch the standing shin stretch. Remain at the rear of a seat and hold the finish of the seat for help and equilibrium. Twist your nails marginally and raise the toes of your feet off the ground while laying behind you. Do this stretch for around 30 seconds.

Hip Stretch

The following one is the hip stretch. Remain at the rear of a seat for help and equilibrium while bowing your nails across and get one lower leg over the inverse leg. Presently sit back, watch and hold it straight for around 30 seconds.

Rehash the stretch, getting the other lower leg over the contrary knee.

Upper back Stretch and shoulder stretch

The following one is the upper backstretch and shoulder stretch. This stretch is ideal for exercises that require the chest area and bowing development. Thus, to start the time, remain behind the seat, and clutch the rear of the seat for help. At that point, remove one stage from the seat until your arms are completely extended. Presently move and twist forward from your midsection and spread your shoulders ahead, at that point, clutch the knee for around 30 seconds.

Attempt to extend however many ways as you can; the more stretches that you do, the more probable, you will be to keep away from tight muscles, forestall wounds, and feel good if your muscles are tight, patient with it. It will require some investment for your muscles to return to their sensible length. Extending for the duration of your life will assist with decreasing the impact of maturing and will assist me with getting thinner and lessen the mileage of your joints and tissue.

Studies have shown that it is feasible to keep up your adaptability through a wide-extending program that you can follow. You ought to recollect that extending isn't a challenge, you shouldn't contrast yourself and others since everyone is unique. Occasionally you may be feeling bar where are a few days you may feel tighter. Stay easily inside your cutoff points and permit the progression of your energy to come through you.

Presently let us look talk about some straightforward activities that will help you during your speculation meeting.

Abs

The first is the abs. Thus, get an air pocket seat or a hand weight and afterward lay your back on it while pointing your feet straight. Take the weight and expand your arms over it, and afterward contract your muscular strength while lifting the load up towards the roof. Breathe out while going up, and breathe in while moving lower. Presently you ought to recall not to bob ready. Moves gradually so your muscles will be tight all through the whole set additionally, attempt to bring your weight at a point and attempt to push the weight straight all completely vertical. Presently the hardware that you need for this activity is hand weights and exercise balls, though the muscles that you are working out are the upper stomach and the center muscles.

Chapter 21 - Self Care Tips and Advice for Eating Better

Self-care is a fundamental part of care and is additionally at the center of keeping up our prosperity. Without it, the remaining sound is inconceivable, and our self-certainty likewise endures. For weight reduction to be useful, and for it to be reasonable, self-care ought to be important for your training.

In any case, what is self-care, precisely?

Characterized as straightforward as could really be expected, this relates to our capacity to take care of ourselves, actually, intellectually, and inwardly. For it to mean something, it should include both the body and psyche. This is particularly valid for individuals who are hoping to build up a better and kinder relationship with themselves, besides basically changing their appearance by getting in shape.

Self-care instructs how to make a supporting relationship with ourselves since this can likewise impact our own decisions and choices. Self-care could spell the contrast between falling back to your old negative routines and forging ahead towards arriving at your objectives since you love yourself an excessive amount to get back to how things were before you began the positive changes.

Through it, we can likewise see a huge decrease in the manner stress influences us. We will start to manage our dissatisfactions identified with flawlessness and blemish. We start to treat ourselves all the more delicately, giving similar energy to people around us, accordingly creating a circle that is brilliant with inspiration and love. One little demonstration of extremist self-love that establishes a climate of help and cares, the very things that individuals who are on an excursion of self-advancement need a great deal.

However, self-care without care will, in general, be unfilled.

It's one thing to improve how we treat ourselves genuinely, bettering our cleanliness and preparing. Treating ourselves to kneads on unpleasant days and getting spoiled when we feel down, are on the whole strategies of self-care; however, they can wind up turning out to be shallow activities without the mindfulness that caregivers. Through the training, we acquire further lucidity on the parts of ourselves we disregard.

This incorporates addictions and propensities that presently don't serve us exactly the same things that may be influencing our connections adversely. It likewise occurs frequently that without applying a careful mentality, our self-care routine just fills in as a form of idealism or interruption from the things that we ought to manage. We wind up utilizing it as a method for desensitizing sentiments that are uncomfortable as opposed to going up against them to end the battle.

In light of that, here are a couple of tips on how you can apply care to your #1 self-care schedules:

Practice thoughtfulness towards your body. See, we are a general public that commends being occupied and continually working. Be that as it may, this sort of outlook is hurtful to both our psychological and physical being. To rehearse graciousness towards your body, you need not spend a ton.

You can start by making more opportunities for rest in your timetable and taking care of your body with the sustenance it needs. Preparing a delectable dinner as opposed to getting take out is likewise a form of self-care. Basic yet powerful.

Adding actual work to your routine is additionally a form of thoughtfulness towards your body. In doing this, you are fortifying it and assisting it with delivering any repressed strain that is accumulated from long stretches of being situated in your work area.

Keep in mind, it isn't only your psyche that necessities an outlet, your body expects it to recuperate too.

Practice thoughtfulness towards others in your life

We zeroed in principally on the self, and while there's nothing amiss with that, we should likewise be aware of how we communicate with others. For certain individuals, self-care implies being selfish and putting themselves first, this is OK; however, long you don't do it to the detriment of others. Obviously, how you draw in with everyone around you can likewise impact how you feel about yourself and the world overall.

For instance

Is it safe to say that you are the kind of individual who is exceptionally controlling of others? It very well may be because you need to be seen a specific way or because you need things to be perfect for you, however this sort of mentality just varieties dissatisfaction and superfluous pressure. The truth is, it is extremely unlikely for you to control or make an individual think as per how you need them to, except if you maneuver them toward doing as such. Obviously, as I'm certain you definitely know, control is something awful to do.

In being thoughtful to others, you likewise surrender any assumptions and demands that trouble you. Simultaneously, you additionally let go of the should be seen a specific path or to be valued in the manner you wish they would.

153

Without these things secure you, you likewise become more liberated and presently don't have to feel the antagonism coming from these sentiments.

Spoil yourself with positive and adoring Affirmations

Today, at whatever point somebody discusses self-care, it normally relates to getting spoiled, for example, going to the spa, getting rubs, putting on a face cover, or going home to relax for individual upkeep. It additionally incorporates the act of legitimate prepping and being aware of one's cleanliness. While every one of these individual "customs" is fundamental, they can likewise be made more powerful by adding Affirmations to each activity.

How? Indeed, for instance:

Utilize cherishing affirmations at whatever point you deal with your skin. "You are gleaming" or "You are kissed by the sun" are only a couple of models. This is particularly if you are having an unpleasant day concerning your appearance.

Perhaps you've, as of late, had, in essence, changes that made you break out or turn out to be more swollen, while you realize that these things will ultimately pass and your body will get back to business as usual, it very well may be difficult for certain individuals to manage it. Thusly, it is simply correct and beneficial to help yourself and be forgiving to remember these progressions simultaneously. Other adoring affirmations you can utilize while doing self-care incorporates:

- "I'm delicate, and that is my solidarity."
- "My body transmits light."
- "My hair will sparkle like the crown that it is."

154

- "My skin will be better, and I will keep on focusing on it."
- "I love each bend of my body."
- "I will keep on supporting myself, inside and outside."
- "My face will emanate the delight I presently feel."
- "My skin will be splendid and clear."
- "I won't let how I feel about my body today influences my energy."
- "I'm pretty much as delightful as how I feel inside."
- "I will wear my garments with certainty today."
- "I will put on my make-up without stressing what others may say."
- "I put resources into items that will help cause me to feel much more certain."
- "I love my body as it is today."
- "I will eat food that is feeding and will help make my body far better."
- "I'm appreciative for my body and how it upholds me consistently."
- "How my body looks today won't characterize how I feel."
- "I'm comfortable and certain about my skin."
- "I won't contrast myself with the glorified pictures I am being taken care of."
- "My body's excellence isn't characterized by another person's assessment of it."
- "I'm appealing, and the assessment of a couple of won't change that."

- "Food isn't my adversary. I will appreciate and give appropriate food to my body."

As usual, these are only a couple of instances of affirmations you can use in the first place. In proceeding with this excursion, you will learn, find, and have the option to make more customized affirmations that take into account your particular necessities.

Keep in mind, the key is to make it enabling and motivating. Regardless of how long or short your affirmations you are, the fact of the matter is that it should leave you feeling sure and fit for accomplishing anything.

Developing New Mini-Habits for Better Eating

A fundamental piece of self-care is contemplating what you devour day by day.

Posing basic inquiries, for example:

- Is this giving me the supplements I need?
- Is this sustaining my body without limit?
- Is this useful for my well-being?

Are basic factors in keeping up, your weight reduction progress, yet your general prosperity also. Be that as it may, these aren't the solitary things you need to zero in on. Your eating propensities are likewise important to the interaction, beginning from purchasing, cooking, setting a plate, and at last eating the food you have arranged. If you apply care to each progression of assembling a dinner, you can give sustenance to the body, brain, and soul.

So, here are a few small propensities you should attempt to create and remember for your ordinary supper time schedule.

Make a careful kitchen

What's the significance here? Regardless of whether you have a full kitchen or even a little washroom in a common residence or condo, its fundamental part would be its substance. Perhaps the most widely recognized reasons with regards to why individuals forego cooking are because they don't have the fixings and the instruments to amplify the time, they have accessible. Ask yourself, how energized will you be to set up a feast on the off chance that you discover that you need a large portion of the fixings and you have no appropriate pots or container to take care of business?

You'll simply wind up requesting take-out, isn't that so?

This is the reason developing a careful kitchen is gainful with regards to eating better and sustaining your body. In doing this, you establish an inviting and quiet climate for you to set up your food in. A spot in your home that sets you in the correct state of mind and makes you eager to cook for yourself and your family. It need not be extravagant, yet it needs to have every one of the nuts and bolts. It likewise pays to have space for an eating region, so you're not eating in random spots at your own home. Thusly, you can make the most of your food utilizing utensils you like and, around there, where there are no interruptions, like the TV. You'll have the option to zero in additional on your eating regimen and on the way toward eating it. On the off chance that you live with others, you can utilize this chance to chat with them more, being at the time all while giving your body the correct sort of food it needs: great home-prepared food, adoring organization, and invigorating discussion.

157

Chapter 22 - Types of Diets to Lose Weight Raw Food Diet

This eating routine is generally clear as crystal. The rules are straightforward: eat just raw foods. Numerous individuals trying to stick to this eating routine slowly bring regular foods into their typical eating regimen until they feel comfortable with a totally raw eating routine. And when we say characteristic, that is stringently what we mean.

These are uncooked and natural foods. No lack of hydration or protection except for raw, new foods, often not prepared with salt. While the dietary benefit isn't far from being obviously true, the raw eating routine can be somewhat restricting.

You will require reliable admittance to new foods and would normally think that it's tough to eat with companions who aren't sticking to a raw eating regimen. This design is likely the toughest to maintain with minimal measure of choices accessible.

Smoothies and servings of mixed greens rule this eating regimen. It is tough to fill yourself in raw foods effectively, also it tends to be expensive to supply since it is only new foods from one day to another. This eating regimen goes about as an incredible method to purge and try different things with, however infrequently, it is drilled for deep-rooted periods beside a minority of individuals.

Paleo Diet

The paleo diet has seen extremely certain reactions from weightlifting networks, just as those looking for a segment of food that is wealthy in social history. The paleo diet depends on what we currently accept that our ancestors ate during agrarian times. These were the occasions before farming saw a lot of meat being devoured, just as raw nuts, seeds, and berries. Some may even feel slanted to forage for the foods or chase for their meat sources.

Logical investigations show understanding into these occasions, proposing that our ancestors were extremely dynamic and basically kept a generally raw eating routine, and all the more strangely, may have abstained during seasons of ineffective chases or forages.

There is a typical misinterpretation that prehistoric man ate only meat.

This is easy to refute, yet most of the specialists propose that the irregularity of chases and enormous clan size would imply that not exactly 50% of the eating regimen would comprise meat. This could shift altogether in various locales of the world, and with the strange idea of our past, it is tough to propose how our ancestors lived precisely. We can securely accept that they ate an eating regimen high in protein and fiber, with insignificant caloric admission, here we see that this idea fits pleasantly into discontinuous fasting rehearses.

While the paleo diet has differing ways of thinking individual to individual, the design is really reliable. Although pinpointing the specific food of past ages is a doomed undertaking, we can give a free rule for what is today thought to be a paleo diet. It is as per the following:

- Lean meats and seafood

- Eggs

- Root vegetables

- Seeds

- Oils like olive or coconut

- Herbs

This is certainly not a far-reaching list; however, a strong fledgling's manual for beginning to work with a paleo-style diet. Remember, these fixings would be wild-foraged or caught and chased upon the arrival of utilization. The fresher the segment, the closer to an authentic paleo diet it is. There are additionally numerous foods stayed away from by disciples of the paleo diet. Consider that horticulture and cultivating wouldn't have existed, such countless foods that are accessible and mainstream in our general public today would not be open. A few models include:

- Legumes

- Grains

- Dairy Products

- Processed oils

- Prepared sugars

- Any handled or frozen foods

Entire Thirty Diet

Ascending in prevalence as of late with the numerous determinations of celiac and other gluten intolerances, the total thirty diets expects one to surrender foods that are regular sensitivities for some individuals. The possibility that these foods are the reason for people building up the hypersensitivities is at the core of this eating regimen.

These foods are viewed as unwanted for followers of this eating routine.

The act of this eating routine itself asks that you do 30-day clean eating, cutting out these unwanted foods to check whether you feel observably better because of intense sensitivity to these normal guilty parties. The suppers often rejected are as per the following:

- Peanuts
- Beans
- Grains, even sans gluten grains
- Other wellsprings of gluten
- Shellfish
- Dairy
- Soy
- Nuts
- Seeds

This rundown is positive does exclude each hypersensitivity causing food. On the off chance that you speculate a supper might be causing destructive responses, cut it out during the spotless eating cycle and see what occurs. Upon steadily presenting these foods, you can observe your body's reactions or scarcity in that department.

The entire thirty diets are an astounding eating regimen for rehearsing consciousness of our bodies. This eating regimen can assist us with building up our abilities and propensities for tuning into our bodies. By independently once again introducing foods after a sort of purifying, we can better figure out how particular sorts of foods respond when we ingest them. This makes the entire thirty eating regimen ideal for planning for irregular fasting. Start the whole thirty eating routine around one month

162

before a fasting week to slip into the IF attitude and make your body for dietary changes.

Vegan Diets

Plant-based diets are extraordinarily mainstream in light of the web and globalization, yet in addition, numerous societies have supported a plant-based standard for centuries. Vegetarianism has seen extraordinary achievement in transforming people for the better; it is broad all through the world, including more than a fifth of the whole populace.

Numerous individuals are pulled into vegan diets to help balance the western world's dependence on meat and creature items. Cultivating businesses add to a significant part of the world's contamination and deforestation issues, in this way, with its medical advantages and biological mindfulness, vegetarianism goes about as a sound eating routine to transform yourself on the individual level and your encompassing world.

Veggie lover rules are easy to follow. You fundamentally do exclude any meat from your eating routine. This could mean a wide range of things to various individuals. A few groups reject meat itself however, eat eggs and utilize creature-based stocks. Different vegans reject any creature items, so no dairy, soups, milk, or eggs. This stricter eating regimen can verge a vegetarian diet, yet veganism will, in general, be tougher, advancing basic entitlements activism.

Veggie lover diets typically incorporate cheeses and dairy, yet it would be on just certain events.

The veggie lover diet is high for the individuals who need a straightforward change to improve their food, and a few groups pick one day of seven days to every vegan; others investigate the menu altogether, often taking in the eating propensities for the remainder of their lives. Vegan fixings would resemble the accompanying rundown:

- Fruits
- Berries
- Dairy
- Eggs
- Beans

Veggie lover Diet

Embracing a veggie-lover diet is like a vegan one; just vegetarians are rigorously plant-based. It does exclude any creature items whatsoever. No dairy, no stocks, no eggs, nectar, and not in any event, utilizing make-up or wearing garments made of creature items. We see here that this eating routine comes outfitted with a way of thinking. Creature activism is an urgent part of veganism. Numerous veggie lovers fight the cultivating business and even censure the taming of creatures.

Vegetarian diets would resemble this:

- Strict no creature utilization
- Vegetables
- Whole Grains
- Berries
- Soy or Tofu

Mediterranean Diet

This eating regimen has a rich history and social explicitness, offering a vivacious course of events and reliable food where the achievement is seen all through every one of the way of life in the Mediterranean district. The positive and celebratory nature of the eating experience in these societies is known all through the world. This is the reason numerous movements to these locales basically to eat and appreciate life. Individuals in the Mediterranean district are strolling instances of the advantages of a charming eating routine and food experience. A Mediterranean shopping rundown may appear to be like this:

- Fruits
- Legumes
- Vegetables
- Fresh Fish
- Olive Oil

The lean, low-calorie, and high-fat substances of this eating regimen make for a reasonable eating routine that adjusts well with a discontinuous fasting schedule. The relationship we work with our bodies ought to be charming and bold, pick a night to set up a Mediterranean gala joined by a red wine from the area to split away from your standard daily practice.

Ketogenic Diet

However, the actual food merits some additional consideration as the eating regimen ascends in prevalence in wellbeing circles. We need to emphasize the risks implied with prompting a deliberate condition of ketosis. If you are thinking about this sort of diet, make certain to do your examination and tune in to your body. We should examine the ketogenic diet in more detail.

Diets that cling to a ketogenic structure are not commonly drilled by fledglings in the irregular fasting networks. The food is viewed as a further developed design than other well-known diets. These diets are by and large high in fat and low in sugar content. Entire grains and bread are stayed away from. Some mandatory foods would be:

- Eggs
- Avocados
- Fatty meats
- Fish

The thinking for this eating regimen comes from the study of ketosis. By restricting caloric admission and diminishing the fast energy we get from sugars and carbs, our bodies will consume stored fat cells as another option. Fat cells are cleaner and more productive energy too; this is the reason we see a lot of fats in a ketogenic diet. We can see here how ketogenic states are instigated through a kind of irregular quick. Forever, you quick from caloric admission and arrive at a condition of ketosis. This is an extremely particular response that the body is outfitted with, going about as an endurance intuition of the most developed form.

Chapter 23 - Nourishing Your Love with Food

Can a sentiment with food appear to be something heartfelt and delectable, or does this seem like a head-on crash with fat addition? What sort of relationship do you like to have with food and eating? In your connections, you will discover two other options: you can choose to keep a relationship with an individual, or you could choose to become "unmarried" or "unattached." Even if another person decides to keep a relationship with you, you have the decision to fall or spill over.

You don't have that decision with ingesting. You can't eliminate yourself from eating and food any huger than you can limit breathing and air out of your life. Since the time you have your dinners can't settle on the choices about its association with you, at that point, you need to make the choice. You can't get away from it. This inquiry will stay substantial: what sort of relationship do you like to have with food and eating? We as a whole know individuals who advise us they would rather not eat and think that it's an issue to make a big deal about it, liking rather have a pill if you were accessible. Plus, we realize the individuals who don't have a cooker and don't have any intention to cook or skill. We all have the opportunity to pick what association they'd love to have with suppers. But since you're perusing this distribution, plainly, individuals share something for all intents and purposes. Like individuals, you may love to devour and wish to savor the food. We can pick to entertain ourselves with an enthusiastic sentiment with food and make the most of our optimal weight.

You Can Eat anything you desire and Maintain Your Perfect Weight

At sixty years of age, we (the essayists) find that we're ready to eat anything we desire and keep up our optimal weight. This limit shows up more genuine for us than different things. We should rehash this, as it catches the core of our association with dinners. We could eat whatever we need, cherishing every single, furthermore, keep up our optimal weight. It's precise to individuals, and it could likewise be sensible for you.

It Appears That Way, so It's That Way

It is how It's finished. By creating a healthy way of life and an association with our dinners, which produces the results or ideal weight we might want, it seems like we could eat anything we desire and keep up our optimal weight.

If no doubt approach individuals, it's veritable for us. It's our fact. It's a reality we are living in. In any case, assuming you investigate our way of life and association with food, you may see that we tune in to that which we purchase, cook, and eat, so we get the results we want. We're continually adjusting our way of life so we could eat anything we desire and keep up our optimal weight. Not only do we settle on reasonable choices about food (a lot of new natural products, organic products, vegetables, and entire grains), we eat sensible part measures, so we as a whole move our bodies; additionally, there are numerous foods that we don't eat since they make undesirable results. Basically: We focus on making a way of life that creates the outcomes we need for a solid and glad body, which is our optimal weight. In this way of life, we're perfectly changed into the traditions and schedules which advantage us with this healthy, glad human body. Our way of life is to be sure compensating that we venerate this, and to us, it shows up as though we could eat whatever we need and revel in our optimal weight. On the off chance that we could do as such, you do as well. An incredible piece of our life spins around dinners, and we may eat more and love eating significantly more than we can right now since we do it with no regret or undesirable feelings. We don't express that these things to brag or gap ourselves from you, yet rather so you will notice you may appreciate a way of life where it seems you could eat what you might want and have your optimal weight. What we recommend is certainly not a weight watcher's or restricted eater's way of life in any capacity. It is a caring relationship with suppers and eating.

You Make It Happen

Karma isn't engaged with getting a sound, cherishing relationship with dinners or different things. In any case, as anyone who's experienced passionate feelings for comprehends, there's specific sorcery to become in a relationship. There's a sorcery that spotlights your energy and uses your enthusiasm to overcome any obstruction capably. The strength of enchantment that makes this happen is on your choices about what you would like, or what moves you, whatever you decide to think, and what you expect.

As we referenced in the stage, every one of these major fixings makes different things happen on your realities; to your optimal weight, this infers reasonable food decisions, work out, and a way of life that creates the outcomes that you want.

Another factor in your relationship with food is the aim and core interest.

169

"Expectation" is a mental thought regarding what you might want. "Care" is the energy or spotlight you put on the thing you're doing. This will furnish you with the result which you might want. As a case, you intend to eat simply enough to be full instead of overstuffed. Your emphasis focuses on biting each chomp carefully, slowly, and finding if the body has had sufficient food. A solid and adoring relationship needs your objective and your thoughtfulness regarding make the results that you might want.

To sustain your unadulterated sentiment with eating and food, let us take a gander at the equal into a solid marriage or association. Hold on for us, for you will track down a couple of very supportive tips which you can attract upon to your relationship with eating and food. On your relationship with suppers, we'll basically inspect the parts of the decision, including homogamy, complementarity, and certainty.

These are exactly the same ideas or blockers included with a solid, profitable relationship or association. Regardless, we'd love to interest the standard of "private propinquity" that says what or who is closest to you, have a greatly improved chance for decision. Or, on the other hand, basically, you're more prone to meet and begin to look all starry-eyed at somebody near you than with somebody who dwells around there, another country, or an alternate country. Similarly, privately developed foods are less difficult to love. Privately developed foods are more delicious and keep up expanded supplement energy contrasted with food that has been grown 3,000,000 miles off and prepared to persevere through an extremely long outing and furthermore to get a long timeframe of realistic usability. Select what's close to your foods which come from any place you dwell. Ranchers' business sectors are among those relational arrangers on your sentiment with food.

Homogamy

One channel in making a relationship involves homogamy, which connotes comparable qualities and interests. You're more disposed to meet and fall head over heels for an individual on the off chance that you yell with people who share similar qualities and interests.

For example, if you like craftsmanship exhibitions, you're more prone to find an amicable companion if you try out a workmanship course contrasted with on the off chance that you yell with people in a seashore volleyball challenge. The equivalent goes for suppers. On the off chance that you'd like your optimal weight, you're bound to achieve that point on the off chance that you encircle yourself with foods which energize solid fat, as new vegetables and products of the soil grains, rather than with foods which aren't viable with your optimal weight, similar to doughnuts, pizza, just as fries.

As seeing someone whom you track down that someone else appreciates the things which you appreciate, you may consider your to be with suppers as a shared interest among you and your dinners. You love the foods that provide you with ideal muscle versus fat, wellbeing, energy, and energy, and these foods affectionately support you and furthermore your physical make-up. By eating foods you appreciate, and which are solid, you may have a great time eating newly.

Complementarity

That is the channel where the contrasts between companions improve the association. The distinctions that you bring into the relationship are currently ready to serve each other's prerequisites and make the association more solid. In an endeavor, it could be the one life partner likes to perform yard work, and others despise it.

One jumps at the chance to manage the financing, cover off the bills, and furthermore compose the tests, while another mate gets a stomachache while the person sees the cash fly from their financial records each month. The distinctions match the mates since everybody serves the prerequisites of another. On your sentiment with suppers, you can permit your dinners to offer you protein, fats, and minerals, which you can't make yourself. Furthermore, therefore, you furnish your dinners with the body movements that consume off the calories and convert that hidden food energy to some meanders through a delightful park.

Your supper gives you an orchestra of heavenly bites and joys.

During your rest days, the human body assimilates the supplements through absorption to get solid tissues, energy, and energy. The following morning, you essentially take your own body to get a walk or to a yoga class or offer it an exercise which moves the burned through supplements to any place they are currently ready to give you the ideal weight which you might want, seeing what colossal advantages food supplies can improve your relationship with dinners.

Whenever that you're eating, consider how much the dinners will feed the human body, alongside your optimal weight.

Chapter 24 - Slimming Secrets to Jump Start Your Extreme Weight Loss

Endermologie

Endermologie is the drug spa method that separates fat cells, permitting fat to be flushed out of your framework, along these lines streamlining the presence of cellulite and banishing it for great. It doesn't do any harm. Plus, it's been logically demonstrated to be just about as much as 200% more compelling than a manual back rub for delivering developed toxins and lactic corrosive.

What to Do

To get more top to bottom data on what causes cellulite, and furthermore explicit procedures that you can expect in an endermologie meeting, tune in to my Instant Audio Seminar, "Hollywood's Best-Kept Anti-Cellulite Secret: Everyone's Doing It, and No One's Talking About It," here:

Detox

No additional bulging food varieties! Avoid broccoli and Brussels grows, and select asparagus, all things being equal! Additionally, you need to drink citrus water with lemon or lime.

What to Do

Opt for purifying food sources like melon, pineapple, watermelon, and honeydews. Likewise, don't belittle the force of espresso.

It's a characteristic diuretic. On the off chance that you are delicate to caffeine, have it in the first part of the day. On the off chance that you need a more solid diuretic, take a preposterous water-shed pill to assist you with killing abundance water weight and "pee off the pounds."

Avoid Sodium

You may be confused by the prospect of soy sauce being sans calorie, believing it's OK to use as a fixing in your eating regimen; in any case, soy sauce is one of the greatest sodium-conspires available. This implies even a touch can prompt a gigantic five-pound gain of water weight.

Additionally, your hands and feet can turn out to be extremely swollen, alongside apparently recognizable puffiness of the neck, jaw, and under-eye territory. It can take a decent 3 to 5 days for your body to cleanse the actual impacts of what soy sauce can do. Soy additionally raises your estrogen levels. Furthermore, don't be tricked by light soy sauce; the sodium content is still high!

Olives are heart-solid, yet in addition, among the most noteworthy sodium-content things on the market, along these lines setting off hunger for fluids, which just adds more water-weight acquire! Pickles are identical in the sodium substance of a sack of potato chips! A scramble of vinegar is certifiably not a genuine vegetable, it is just a cucumber that has been absorbed in sodium and additives! Attempt to stay away, olives and pickles. Simply evaporate you and get dried out! Yuck! If you must have an olive, wash off the additional sodium.

On the off chance that you are attempting to lean out in 7 days, ensure you avoid peanut butter, nuts, cheddar, and diet pop, alongside the entirety of the other clear food sources that you would not devour on the off chance that you are consuming fewer calories.

What to Do

Opt for salt-and without sodium flavors like Mrs. Run. Decide on a tablespoon of olive oil to receive the wellbeing rewards of olives, in addition to its extraordinary for your hair, skin, and nails. On the off chance that you get a hankering for pickles, pick cucumbers, or other precut vegetables with a low-sodium salad dressing.

Try not to Eat Carbs after 4 P.M.

Try not to eat carbs after 4 p.m. It flabbergasts me how often I have heard from ladies in the entirety of my discussions, which were all the while eating carbs after 4 p.m. furthermore, hoping to get in shape. I heard so often that they were devouring pasta, potatoes, slices of bread, rice, and furthermore moves at supper, and they couldn't comprehend why their weight was not moving.

What to Do

Aim not to eat complex carbs after your late-evening nibble.

You should have a carb at breakfast and for your midmorning nibble, of course at lunch, and afterward again with your late-evening feast. The significant standard to recall here isn't to have a carb at supper on the grounds that, thusly, you will be working with your digestion as opposed to against it. The science is unadulterated. On the off chance that you do eat a carb around evening time, you might be storing it on your body, and afterward, your body should work more enthusiastically in the first part of the day to consume it off. I encourage you to figure out how to "work more efficiently" toward your weight-loss objectives. By eating a protein and a stringy carb at supper (for instance, a flame-broiled chicken bosom, a green plate of mixed greens, and a serving of steamed asparagus), you will lay out the groundwork for yourself the following day when you are working out, with fewer carbs to consume off!

Exercise in the Morning

Try not to misunderstand me; exercising whenever of the day is acceptable! It has its medical advantages; be that as it may, to get the most outcomes and to get more fit all the more rapidly, you should attempt to work out in the mornings. Practicing around evening time can some of the time meddles with your standard dozing designs given the spike of energy you get from applying energy so late in the day.

What to Do

It has been experimentally demonstrated that the first thing toward the beginning of the day is the ideal opportunity to work out because it jump-starts your digestion!

Jump Rope

It's been demonstrated that only 10 minutes of jumping rope is what might be compared to running for 60 minutes! It is additionally an exceptionally convenient exercise with the goal that you can do it anyplace!

What to Do

Coming up next is a proposed schedule that will assist you with maximizing your jump-rope exercise and have some good times doing it: Tan Utilize self-leather experts! You can really "tan off" around five great pounds! All wellness models and those in the wellness business depend on this proprietary advantage. They realize that the body looks less fatty and more toned with a more obscure skin tone.

Moreover, your teeth seem whiter, and your skin appears flaw-free when you are tan. Having a tan smooth out skin break-out stains, stretch imprints, and the presence of cellulite.

Chapter 25 - The Weight Loss Struggle Cycle

How goes it with you? I trust the Weight Struggle has given you a superior comprehension of the components that are making your weight struggle. Presently I might want to put those components together and walk you through the weight struggle cycle. This baffling and self-disrupting cycle epitomizes the hardware of restricting convictions, propensities, and feelings and is controlled by the inner critic and inner rebel.

The weight struggle cycle gives us that disappointing sensation of being caught in this win or bust, fortunate or unfortunate, an on-or-off-a-diet cycle that causes us to feel like we are in this ceaseless un-carousel with respect to weight.

Investigate the cycle on the grounds that soon you will figure out how to get away from its jail. For you to keep away from it, you need to realize how the period functions.

The weight struggle cycle is broken into two stages:

- The "Being Good" Phase
- The "Being Bad" Phase

These stages can be separated into a succession of steps that get worked out on a psyche level.

The weight struggle cycle: The "Being Good" Phase

Here we are at the highest point of the weight struggle cycle. It generally starts as the weight struggler rises up out of a being terrible period of going off course and indulging.

Stage 1: The Initial Impulse to Lose Weight

The initial phase in the cycle is the routine "I need to get more fit!" response to feeling a negative feeling. The trigger to that undesirable inclination can be outer or inside, for example:

- The number on the scale.

- Somebody says something regarding your weight.

- You have a liberal few days of indulging and drinking.

- A specialist's admonition.

- Understanding a wedding or gathering or the seashore season is occurring soon.

Stage 2: Find Some Method to Lose Weight ASAP

This following stage includes tracking down a fast answer to get us out of the agony of feeling overweight or crazy and in the driver's seat once again. This sort of reasoning makes us helpless against outrageous eating regimens or other weight-loss strategies (diets, scrubs, practice systems, or pills) to get the weight off. Frequently, we never truly stop to think if the procedure is sound from a well-being point of view or is sensible for our way of life.

One customer trusted me: "If you gave me a container of soil and some water and said I would shed 20 pounds simply by eating it, I would have done it to lose the weight and escape that spot of agony!"

Stages 3: Start a Diet and Feel in Control for a While

This progression in the cycle may continue for quite a long time, days, weeks, or even months if the weight struggler gets into a "being awesome" groove. There may likewise be a sort of diet high, that is, an inclination of being in charge, large and in charge!

Hooray! However long the eating routine and exercise system goes easily, the inner critic is calm and offers acclaim for the "great" conduct. Also, as long as the scale continues to go down, everything is great in the fat reasoning world.

Stage 4: Willpower Fades

The following stage in the cycle happens when the will to keep up the eating regimen or exercise plan debilitates, as it does in circumstances like these: The weight struggler feels denied of old propensities and delight.

- The weight struggler can't eat what every other person is eating.
- The eating routine is excessively prohibitive and difficult to follow.
- The scale quits going down, and the weight struggler doesn't have the foggiest idea why.
- Stress and life responsibilities meddle.

Indeed, even momentary triumphs like these can challenge the weight struggler: The weight struggler loses some weight and fits once again into clothes.

Others say the weight struggler looks great.

The weight struggler arrives at an all the more reasonable number on the scale.

For this situation, the agony that drove the weight struggler to eat less has blurred.

Therefore, his determination to remain on the part of food begins to lessen too.

With either of these situations, the weight struggler moves rapidly to Step 5.

Stage 5: Going Off "Being Good"

Someplace in the "being acceptable" stage, as resolution or resolve lessens, the weight struggler will definitely eat some "awful food" (that food being whatever the weight struggler's inner critic considers is forbidden.) The blast of sugar and fat in the weight struggler's mouth causes a chain response of delight. Maybe firecrackers are detonating in the brain!

The quick-thinking part about the mind kicks right into it, and the telephone begins ringing again for a greater amount of the stuffing food. It doesn't take well before the delight of getting a charge out of the food offers a path to the inner critic's disgracing reprimands. "Take a gander at what you did! You were doing so well, and you blew it!"

Stage 6: Feeling Bad

It's disturbing to feel like we have blown it when attempting to eat less. Then the need to look for cover from the Inner-Critic-initiated sensations of blame and disgrace emerges. That upsetting ringing telephone of propensity presently expects and needs a greater amount of the swelling and soothing food, leaving an ideal opening for the Inner Rebel to step in and start his temptation.

The Weight Struggle Cycle: The "Being Bad" Phase

There are a couple of essential minutes between the "Being Good" stage and the "Being Bad" stage. In this short, however, fundamental time, we have a decision to refocus or surrender. Weight Masters will stop, calmly inhale, and refocus. This is the way to consistency and weight authority. (You will figure out how to do this soon, I guarantee!) Weight strugglers proceed onward to Step 7.

Stage 7 Screw It, Start over Tomorrow

This is the most well-known propensity that is wired into the Weight Struggler's brain.

There's a practically prompt positive feeling at being off the eating regimen snare and having the permit to eat without blame and disgrace.

The more occasions the Weight Struggler tumbles off an eating regimen, the more the "I blew it, so screw it!" reaction is supported in the Weight Struggler's brain, making the cycle practically difficult to stay away from. The joy in the delivery and help from the limitation of the eating regimen is verifiable. The issue is the thing that continues in the subsequent stage.

Stage 8 Eat: with Reckless Abandon

The eating train has left the station and is pushing ahead with the amazing propensity for "eat around evening time since tomorrow is hardship day!"

Without even completely encountering the flavor of food or its underlying delight, the weight struggler allows oneself to eat "whatever," which typically implies whatever food varieties have been forbidden.

Then, after the inner rebel is satisfied from eating all that awful food and is sluggishly sitting in the corner, the inner critic awakens, invigorated, and prepared to welcome the real world. The weight struggler currently feels regretful and restless about being so wild and reboots the cycle.

For what reason, DOES BEING BAD FEEL SO GOOD?

So, you ate something you shouldn't have and ruined you're eating plan?

You guarantee to begin once again tomorrow, and out of nowhere, you feel incredible! Here are a few reasons why:

1.   The guarantee for future goodness acquits present disagreeableness. At the point when our psyche expects our being valuable later on (like going on an exacting eating routine Monday), the synapse dopamine floods our brain and causes us to feel better. To us, we feel temperate as though we were at that point charming although it's Sunday night and we are finishing that last cut of pizza!

2.   You get the disturbing ringing telephone of "begin once again tomorrow." Recall your old companion propensity and how a signal, similar to a ringing telephone, triggers the desire to get it? "Feeling terrible" goes about as a trigger that forces us to "begin once again." Pretty precarious, huh? Very much like getting the telephone brings help from the disturbance of the ringing, the psychological missteps the sensation of solace for delight or unwinding.

3.   You will break the obligations of a prohibitive eating routine and eat anything you desire! When encircled by enticing high-fat, sweet food sources, you may feel a huge rush of extra excitement as your pleasure synapses become invigorated. Dr. David Kessler, in his book The End of Overeating, calls this wonder "hyper-incitement."

Chapter 26 - Additional Tips to Help You Lose Weight

How, if there's one thing numerous individuals are as yet managing on the planet today, its pointless weight acquires, which is set off by too much cheap food.

Be that as it may, with the guide of your side's wellness book and a couple of thoughts you can test, you will altogether diminish your body's abundance of fat to give you a youthful look you've had previously.

While it is an interaction that takes some time, if you need to dispose of your new body position by any means, you, as the person in question, will show a lot of determination just as control. Also, what is a portion of the stunts with the wellness manual close by that will cause you to lose weight inside the briefest measure of time?

The main thing you can work out is to eat a lot of products from the soil and limit fat-rich food sources.

Having that at the top of the priority list, you ought to have a subsequent routine practice that you can do, including going for a short walk, on the off chance that you think that it's difficult to perform thorough exercises. This will urge you to eat extremely adjusted food sources and do a couple of light wellness manual activities from the manual.

The other counsel is to practice good eating habits, natural suppers, which will contain more vegetables and organic products, and drink green tea after each inspiring dinner you take. This strategy is extremely effective, explicitly for the individuals who favor thinning down the common way.

Less calorie admission would likewise essentially help to diminish the body weight because too numerous calories in the body start to hinder the body's metabolic cycle, accordingly adding to the weight previously acquired.

This is one troublesome choice that numerous individuals may not be adequately thoughtful to take, yet it is the lone way out of the weighty issue. Also, if you decide to devour less calorie food sources and perform distinctive wellness manual activities, at that point, your imperative body digestion rate will ricochet once more into shape quicker than you anticipated. Did you see that drinking a lot of water will help you lose weight rapidly also?

At the point when you're on an exacting eating regimen to lose weight, the body should be hydrated constantly to keep up its ideal levels and lessen the abundance of weight gain and water maintenance that may be available in the body. You're all set, with a little wellness support. Numerous tips to help you lose weight quicker, incorporate eating potassium-rich food varieties, calcium, routine exercises, utilizing the wellness manual or video, a solid eating regimen plan, and an inspirational perspective all through.

Disregard the anguishing stories you read about the fact that it is so tough to lose weight.

Make it simpler for yourself to help you lose weight by following these 10 speedy and simple tips. Execute one tip each day, and you'll be at your objective weight before you know it: no problem, and there is no compelling reason to flip around your entire world by the same token. Try not to squander any more energy on meds and costly medicines or hard-made money, begin to utilize these tips today and furthermore be lean and sound.

The primary stunt to help you lose weight is to have good dieting propensities. Thusly, you can acquire more food amount; however, you can likewise utilize regular low-calorie flavors like onions to improve the taste. It is known for long-haul prosperity, and weight misfortune as the eating routine weight itself is wiped out.

Cut back the excess consistently off the meats that you cook. Or, on the other hand, if it is chicken-like, cut the excess. Slash it up and add it to something like pasta, if that is too boring!

Get a companion responsible for your eating routine program. Individuals will, in general, be more dedicated following possibly 14 days when they know, and need to check in with others. First off, discover somebody to stroll with, a close companion, or even an eating regimen beau. Say your objectives! In some cases attempting to accomplish something without anyone else can be much harder.

To monitor calories, starches, proteins, and so on, record all that you burn through. You would be stunned if you didn't record your menu, the number of additional things you would drink. Either plan with your dietary admission or begin keeping a food log to see!

Utilizing a non-stick canola cooking shower, on the off chance that you need to broil stuff. It will save you a lot of calories over oil cooking. One tablespoon of cooking oil, for instance, contains 120 calories! Taking into account that a 2.4-second PAM shower contains only 16 calories.

Keep the standpoint idealistic, and never surrender. When/on the off chance that you leave, it is the solitary time you battle. It might take further work or some other methodology; however, it "will" occur. Studies show that most individuals battle to attempt their first time. Nothing will replace assurance! Not astuteness, not ability, totally none! The remainder is auxiliary.

Their eating regimen and health programs are 50/50 accomplices in the weight misfortune program. At the point when either is missing, you'll have less possibility of accomplishment! You can exercise until you drop; however, you would not see intense upgrades in your appearance if you take too numerous calories in. Furthermore, on the off chance that you don't do work out, the body is bound to utilize muscle as opposed to fat for energy. Oxygen-consuming activity causes fat consumption! Appetite consumes fat!

Ponder the deficiency of fat and not simply the general weight misfortune. How important is your size, and not the amount you gauge? You might be astonished because the muscle is more significant than fat! So realize calories ignite with the tissue!

So eat dinners consistently and don't miss it. At the point when you hang tight for over four hours, your digestion will begin easing back down.

Realize where fat seems to get the body. Ladies appear to amass fat around their thighs and gluts. Men acquire it on their guts and around their midsection. This is a result of the absence of dissemination in those areas. Fat isn't taken as fast into the circulation system as in different areas. That is the reason fat-consuming specialists, for example, ephedrine, works close by a drawn-out weight misfortune plan. Help even to blood-diminishing specialists like ibuprofen. In any case, before utilizing any substitution, ensure you read the marks, bearings, and cautions!

Keep your weight misfortune program clear. On the off chance that you begin missing suppers or skipping exercises, it eases back your advancement to the place of debilitation. How awful do you need that to occur? Select and adhere to a decent arrangement. Know, what you put in your receives in return!

The vast majority are getting more aware of their weight, not in light of what it means for how they look, yet in addition given the results of their prosperity. In case you're one of those hoping to get a less fatty body, you unquestionably ought to be engaging the straightforward yet fruitful methods.

Betray the universe of cheap food

Obviously, requesting food from a drive-through or via telephone is looser, yet on the off chance that your heart is set to lose huge weight, this is the initial move towards accomplishing such an objective. You'll need to begin eating at home as an alternative, or in case you're a bustling individual and can't deal with such a task, you can generally eat at cafés that have a sound menu on offer. Walking out on inexpensive food will likewise mean surrendering handled food varieties like firm chips and carbonated beverages.

Apply more fluids to your eating regimen

Water is a critical factor in the weight misfortune cycle since it is the transporter of the relative multitude of supplements from the food you burn through. Remembering this, ensure you drink at any rate eight full glasses of water a day, just as a couple of glasses of new natural product juice. Citrus foods grown from the ground make astounding shakes since they taste awesome, and they contain numerous cell reinforcements too.

Track down the Right Weight Loss Supplement, Though

Some individuals are passionately against utilizing a wide range of weight misfortune helps, for example, fat-decrease tablets, yet having a little lift is not much. In any case, it is basic to pick the right type of supplement and to avoid "convenient solution things" that are presently extremely basic available.

Devote 1 hour out of each day for work out

Designate in any event one entire hour for cardio, regardless of how bustling you are at home or work. If you have home rec center gear, you can create faster outcomes as you can work out day by day. An option is going around your local square each day for a total of 30 minutes to 60 minutes.

Set Realistic Objectives

Never expect too a lot of yourself, and you will not get too disturbed if your arrangements don't work out. The best strategy is to take it each day in turn and let your body change by your new eating regimen and exercise schedule.

As it's all the more broadly known, celiac infection or gluten hypersensitivity is progressively getting more predominant in the industrialized world in which we live.

Weight acquires, and Celiac illness isn't something that goes connected at the hip, with weight misfortune being one of the fundamental factors in Celiac disease. Have you been determined to have gluten intolerance recently, and battled with adding the pounds? Allow me to give you a couple of speedy tips to add to your eating routine to help you shed the additional pounds.

I expressed that weight acquires, and celiac illness isn't for the most part connected with each other; however, that doesn't imply that numerous individuals don't have an issue. The facts demonstrate that out of nowhere, around 99% of individuals will see a sensational weight misfortune, and that can have an astonishing impact on their day-by-day lives.

Weight gain and experiencing Celiac infection. Furthermore, for what reason do I pour on the pounds?

I will attempt to clarify that rapidly and without any problem. It is fundamental to know why you could put on weight so you can step on and dispose of the additional weight in your new way of life. At the point when you change your eating routine into gluten-free things, a considerable lot of these don't have the number of supplements your body needs to perform effectively, and that is a conspicuous issue. You can get worn out, torpid, and you can feel unwell. No development or exercise would imply that you don't lose any calories and that you put on weight.

A portion of different causes, and the essential one for some victims, is the abrupt change in the eating regimen to all the more high-fat food sources. Numerous individuals trust it's in every case low in fat, since an item is sans gluten, and that is not the situation.

Chapter 27 - Common Weight Loss Misconceptions

The universe of wellness is loaded with conceivable speculations that case that it will help you in achieving your targets. Some are significant, while others may bring you down a road of superfluous difficult work and deceiving results. This handles the pervasive misconceptions when using preparing and nourishment to accomplish your body.

Misinterpretation #1: Cardio to Shed Weight

You, much of the time, see people running a lot of miles on the treadmill to thin down. Although cardio upgrades general prosperity, it's not fundamental to have the option to consume off fat. Cardio practices like running, trekking, and the curved machines are apparatuses to help fast weight decrease; however, the deciding variable to if your weight changes are the body's equilibrium of calories. Cardio might be an exercise in futility if you're eating routine isn't under control. Via occasion, someone may run ten mph that consumes off 1,000 calories, at that point devour 1,500 calories and lead to putting on weight. Weight decrease is best cultivated by controlling your eating regimen plan. A banana is typically 100 calories, and it needs around 100 calories to run 1 mile. All in all, could it be less difficult to run a mile or simply not eat a banana? Except if you are a contender and fantasize over bananas, at that point, it would likely be easier to forestall running a mile. This is an excellent instance of getting more astute about accomplishing your objective, as opposed to workaholic behavior yourself. When you're eating regimen is within proper limits, you would then be able to think about oxygen consumption to burn calories.

While cardio supports weight decrease, doing an excess of can frequently represent a cleaned look on your muscles. Weight preparing, then again, builds up your muscles, which adds extra detail to your body.

Use your calories to the activities, which will make the sort of results you want. Although you can get a fabulous body without utilizing cardio, it's advantageous under particular conditions. It could be a serious test to give your body adequate sustenance while clinging to a low-carb diet.

Thus, cardio helps consume additional calories, which can empower you to shun, decreasing the number of calories you eat while endeavoring to dispense with fat.

Misinterpretation #2: Toning

To have the option to acquire a "conditioned" look that numerous individuals need, an individual ought to either decrease their muscle to fat ratio or construct extra muscle. By doing this, you can indicate your body considerably quicker. You may simply make your muscles greater or more modest, and you may just acquire or dispense with fat. Fat can't transform into muscle building, nor will muscle transform into fat. Diminishing your muscle to fat ratio needs you to consume a greater number of calories than you eat. To have the option to build muscle, you need to move your muscles enough to create through the utilization of exercise. A few groups every now and again need to keep an indistinguishable weight while accomplishing a conditioned body. As a pound of tissue is denser than a pound of fat, at that point, it's probably going to get a more characterized body when gauging something very similar. Muscles require significantly more to create than needed to dispose of fat. Hence, your weight will presumably diminish as a result of the decrease of fat when arriving at these results in a short period.

194

Misinterpretation #3: Targeting Fat Loss

A few groups need to shed fat simply in their gut, legs, or another bit of the body. Focusing on the decline in fat in a specific spot in your body isn't doable. The districts where you lose and acquire fat are as of now given by your hereditary qualities. A couple of spaces of fat on the body will take more time to disappear than numerous others. Via case, somebody may lose most of the fat in their arms while as yet holding a lot of fat around their tummy. The lessening in the mid-region is divided between the additional provoking districts to wipe out the fat. To have the option to consume off fat in that difficult area, you may just have to continue to work out. At long last, the body will decide to consume off fat from the obstinate zones once it arrives at a lower extent of muscle versus fat loss. There isn't any activity or material which will cause it feasible for you to consume off fat in one specific locale of the body.

Misinterpretation #4: Abs-Training

A few people today accept that to have extraordinary abs, and you need to instruct them hard day by day. The abs need time to recover precisely like different muscles on the whole body, so instructing them normally isn't essential. Abs best respond to high redundancies and brief rest periods between sets.

Carrying out additional weight on your stomach muscle preparation can help create more noteworthy mass. Ensure that you select activities that will focus on all of their abs, like the upper, lower, and slanted areas. It's significant not to fail to remember that your muscle to fat ratio percent must be adequately little to decide your abs. You can prepare your abs adequately to grow, however on the off chance that you have a thick layer of fat inside the stomach, at that point, they will not be noticeable.

Misinterpretation #5: Eating Junk Food

Eating shoddy nourishment doesn't have to get in the strategy for achieving Your activity target. The more you comprehend how your body handles food, is that the more blame you'll feel about all that you eat. Whatever you eat or drink will likely be rearranged to a carb, fat, or protein. Accordingly, regardless of whether you eat a cheeseburger, nonetheless, you're as yet inside your macronutrient focuses for the afternoon, at that point, you will not upset the improvement of shedding pounds or building muscle.

Along with the IIFYM (If It Fits Your Macros) methodology for shedding weight, we regularly get confounded into trusting you should eat as much shoddy nourishment that you need in as much as it finds a way into your macronutrient goals. Although doing so can allow you to understand your ideal body, your internal wellbeing will be in harm's way. Before conceding to a cheeseburger or milkshake, make certain you are getting most of your sustenance from entire food sources each day.

Misinterpretation #6: Alcohol

Most people are hesitant to drink cocktails in alarm. It will demolish the headway towards their activity objective. It's fine to get some liquor since it's with some restraint. Liquor has calories (7 calories for every gram), hence understanding the sum from the drink and the number of calories you're allowed can help you keep on pace for accomplishing your activity objective. It's feasible to substitute the calories out of drinking to get some fat or starches on this day, yet ensure that you're getting sufficient healthy sustenance from food since liquor will not inventory any.

Carrying out vigorous or extra active work on your program may help consume additional calories to allow space for a refreshment or 2. It's useful to burn through much water ahead to diminish parchedness and abundance drinking.

Having a periodic lager or wine will not jumble up your headway insofar as you can fit it into a healthy eating regimen.

Misinterpretation #7: Too Much Sugar

Burning through much sugar cane, without a doubt, brings about long-haul wellbeing chances like diabetes, organ disappointment, and bunches of sicknesses. Be that as it may, concerning the fat loss, eating extensive amounts of sugar will not hold you back from losing weight, given that the fundamental calories to consume off fat are satisfied after some time. All crabs are separated into sugar once processed from the human body. Some food assets like complex carbs take more time to separate, while some end up being in a direct structure like sugar. Since your whole body utilizes glucose as a basic wellspring of fuel during active work, the more dynamic you're is that the more carbs you're permitted. The individuals who consume numerous calories may take out burning-through more sugar as it's being utilized instead of aggregating in the human body. Sugar has unfavorable criticism as it's not difficult to gorge. Similarly, like whatever else, having a lot of anything could be terrible for you. Devouring entire food sources that can be really filling and nutritious assists with balancing the overall utilization of sugar. Concerning getting more fit, subbing sweet food sources like crude nectar or agave nectar for unadulterated sugar is irrelevant because they actually involve basic carbs that separate to sugar on your framework. Sugars like 'Equivalent,' ' Splenda,' or Stevia will, in any case, affect since they incorporate zero calories. Perceiving the number of carbs, you're allowed can permit you to know about how much sugar you can burn while seeking after your activity target.

Misinterpretation #8: Too Much Sodium

Focusing on your salt utilization assumes an irrelevant part in consuming structures or fat muscle. This is substantially more of a safety measure into your general prosperity as opposed to a prerequisite for building a phenomenal body. Directing measures of sodium may decrease pulse while limiting the threats of cardiovascular illness and stroke. At the point when sodium is in the human body, it follows water and keeps the equilibrium of liquids. Also, it works with potassium to keep up electronic techniques across cell films, and this can be fundamental for neural transmission, muscle compression, and different capacities. The body can't work without sodium, thusly limiting your utilization with no regard to exactly the amount you really want, perhaps a potential danger. An expansion in sodium incites your framework to devour more water, Which is the reason your body weight changes for the duration of the day. Lessening sodium admission will assist with diminishing muscle to fat ratio however is fundamental because of the brief decrease of water. It's important to recollect that, in many occurrences, the goal isn't to kill water but to consume off fat. There are huge examples to screen sodium consumption, for instance, if planning for a working out challenge or photoshoot. Jocks or variants may control their salt utilization to introduce their body a sterile, skin-tight charm when they're sufficiently fit to notice the detail of the muscles.

Chapter 28 - Background Information Required for Weight Loss

You may wind up building up certain propensities without knowing. The equivalent applies to make superb wellbeing practice. Your everyday practices and decisions clarify your present conditions. Quit grumbling; do zero in on your propensities a recollect your inclinations will characterize who you will be. Albert Einstein proceeds to say, "we can't tackle our issues with a similar reasoning we utilized when we made them." Step out of your air pocket a given design for the ideal result. Actually, the hardest part is beginning, and you've effectively done that, and it will just get more available and more regular the more you partake and the more you play a functioning job in this excursion.

Consider propensities improvement as expounded in the account of a Miller and a camel on a colder time of year day. It was freezing outside, and keeping in mind that the mill operator was sleeping, he was stirred by some clamor on the entryway. After opening his eyes, he heard the voice of a camel grumbling that it was cold outside and was mentioning to warm his nose inside. Mill operator concurred that he was distinctly to embed the spout. A little later, the camel put his forehead then the neck, at that point different pieces of the body than the entire body step by step until he began obliterating things inside. He began strolling in the house, staggering on anything on its way. At the point when the mill operator requested the camel to move out, they came flaunted that he was comfortable inside and would not leave. The camel went further to tell the mill operator that he could leave at his pleasure. The equivalent goes for a propensity that comes thumping about and dominating. Perhaps you began smoking your first cigarette, thinking it was sickening, and afterward, years pass by, and you have an awful propensity. All things considered, detrimental routines can sneak in; however, a similar way of thinking can apply to moral practices. Simply take it little by little and bit by bit, and before you know it, you have solid propensities in your day-to-day existence. There are countless difficulties to good dieting. You must have a receptive outlook and reset your deduction on food.

It is less expensive to grow new propensities; effort is the essential necessity, however not excessively much. At the point when you have prepared yourself new examples, train on it consistently for some time, after which it will be programmed. We can relate that circumstance to a football club Coach who participates in different thorough preparations with his players while anticipating the genuine match. They practice new abilities and moves.

At the point when match day shows up, the mentor sits with the substitutes while observing the players playing from the line. Players play according to the mastered abilities and moves. Apply the required effort to realize your objective.

While storying with your coworkers, disclose to them how you drink 3 to 4 glasses of water each day, equivalent to tea. That looks exacting. In heart, you know how your utilization of water and group is decreased while at home.

This is self-control. Self-restraint requires the foundation of solid establishments. Efforts embraced are less.

Apply Core arrangements

Perceive and face the difficulties of good dieting and grow new propensities.

Like a lumberjack attempting to clear a log, recognize the basic side of every circumstance.

The all-around experienced lumberjack will attempt to recognize fundamental joints by moving up then do the clearing. A less experienced lumberjack would begin by the edge.

The two techniques produce anticipated outcomes, yet one way saves additional time and uses less energy than the other. Every one of our issues has vital focuses. What about when we distinguish basic logs from good dieting and offer a few arrangements. To start with, log jam. How you were raised. You may have been forced as a kid to eat vegetables and consider it to be something bothersome, and you assembled a discernment that plants don't taste great. Another log jam is pressure. Such a lot of pressing factors.

We live in a world loaded with pressure where time matters in the entirety of our endeavors, grieved life, and our body address a large portion of the cost. You have numerous decisions to pick from. On the off chance that you are an admirer of inexpensive food, you need to stop. Quick food sources are addictive, and we exceptionally rely upon them because of the uplifting perspective we have towards them. We are fixated on them to such an extent that we can't live a day without devouring them. As per Anitapoems., when you eat something incorrectly for you and you say, you couldn't care less. Your musings and spotlight are absolutely on how delightful and pleasant it is to eat the food that you're eating, paying little mind to how unfortunate it is, and afterward you have blame about how those pounds are going on as opposed to falling off.

Such musings happen in any event when taking delicious food. We may end up eating some food which in all actuality we know are hazardous to our wellbeing.

Chip is a great representation. A person from an eating routine class may feel hungry on her way back home and choose to a branch by an inexpensive food joint for certain plates of chips. Notwithstanding a few alerts on the perils of chips from class exercises, she decides to eat chips, what an extreme thought. The vast majority have

mental issues making it hard to quit taking some food although we comprehend their repercussions on our bodies. i.e., eating chips. An article on this theme guarantees that most food organizations are taking a stab around evening time to make inexpensive food more addictive. As indicated by Howard Moskovitz, an expert in the shoddy nourishment industry, they put more flavor on low-quality nourishment to make you return for additional. Assuming the food tastes excessively great, we'd have what's known as a tangible explicit Satia T, then we wouldn't need any longer. So, organizations need to discover the perfect equilibrium of flavors. So, there's not all that much or excessively little.

Everything they do is adjust the flavors. That equilibrium is called the Bliss point.

As indicated by Steven Weatherly, a specialist in lousy nourishment, Cheetos are the center wellspring of joy. They are the particular kind of food fabricated by enormous organizations to exclusively fulfill you and not to add any medical advantage to your body. They are planned in such a way that when you begin eating them, it dissolves on your mouth, making it feels delectable and noteworthy. They are made to make you go for additional. A companion was previously an eating regimen, and her beau got back Cheetos. Indeed, she said no. She wound up having one, and before she knew it, she knew practically the entire thing. Presently we comprehend why the following log in our manner is possibly we figure we don't care for quality food. Maybe you don't care for good food. You need food sources that energize your sense of taste to feel invigorated, be nearer to something energizing, yet you won't be fulfilled.

You'll not arrive at the most extreme point, and maybe you won't realize what to do. Normalizing detrimental routines cause us to feel comfortable in our negative contemplations. At the point when you do something negative, the impacts broadly spread. Egocentrism keeps us enveloped with this protected spot and keeps us within ourselves and consumed by adverse considerations. You know, you do one thing inadequately or adversely, it streams into different regions. It leaves you feeling terrible, and you improve only for the present moment, for example, inconceivable eating regimens that you can't stay aware of, and afterward you, you feel more awful and more regrettable about yourself and, you go over the edge when you can't keep up. It's an endless loop. The essential technique for conquering these key log is to clench hand, hit the reset button. It probably won't be simple, endeavor however much you can by having a receptive outlook and an uplifting perspective going ahead.

Investigate different flavors regardless of whether you don't care for them. Michael's sister has a negative mentality towards blueberries. She had not burned through any since her youth and continued recounting stories that had no association with the blueberries' taste. One day Michael made her taste the blueberry, and she cherished it. Test your presumptions, test your conclusions since you don't have a clue where they came from; such a suspicion might be outlandish. Despite her reason for blueberries being untidy, and she attempted, and she wound up cherishing it.

Open your brain for novel thoughts. Recollect the tale of the demure, and to keep allegorically hurling yourself in more critical conditions, you will loosen up and fill in size. Embrace a mentality of accomplishment and stop hatchling thinking and realize that your considerations, discernments, and practices can change.

Why not begin to anticipate products of the soil, anyway insane they sound? You were not brought into the world with contemplations you have today; they are a build of your brain. They can be tested.

The following arrangement calls for changing one's wellbeing. Saying a major NO and breaking a cycle is all you need, removing guilty pleasure. Submit yourself every day, and you'll see it simpler to conquer the thought of food businesses that need you to be dependent on their food. The third is the development of what you need and the opportunity you want. This progression calls for extraordinary consistency.

Make your striking stage an example. This example will form into the ideal propensity. Unload your actual self through profound confidence and thoughtful quiet.

Endeavor to turn out to be better. A glimpse inside quit searching for arrangements outwardly. Put forth extra attempts like being more useful to those that are glad and really focusing on those that are destitute, reliably go after truth, effortlessness, and harmony in your day. Take alert on taking care of the business of individuals, and you might be carrying on with an off-putting life. At long last, frameworks create self-rule. We will be making a framework together by arranging, keeping it basic, accepting equilibrium in your life, and achieving these arrangements and your objectives by following the framework to assist you with focusing on and reinforce consistency in your life.

The best answer for weight loss is a sound eating regimen and a functioning body. There could be a motivation behind why doing these two is an issue from your side. The pathway will make the interaction more comprehensive and more fun. It may not be your answer, however, you should get something from it.

Chapter 29 - What to Eat and Avoid

The rundown of occasional food varieties to quick ought to include:

For Protein

The Recommended Dietary Allowance (RDA) is 0.8 g of protein per kg of body weight for protein. In light of your wellbeing objectives, just as the degree of movement, the necessities can vary. By decreasing energy utilization, expanding satiety, and improving digestion, protein causes you to shed pounds. Expanded protein utilization creates muscle when combined with strength preparation. Getting further muscle in the body builds digestion since a greater number of calories are consumed by the tissue than fat. A new investigation shows that getting more muscle in your legs may assist with lessening the development of stomach fat in sound men.

The IF protein food list incorporates:

- Poultry and fish
- Eggs
- Seafood
- Yogurt, milk, and cheddar items
- Seeds and nuts
- Beans just as vegetables
- Soya
- Whole grains

For Carbohydrates

45 to 65 % of your calories should come from carbs (starches), as indicated by the American Dietary Guidelines. Carbs are the body's essential fuel source. The other two are fats and proteins. Starches come in various structures. Sugar, fiber, just as starch, is the most huge. Carbs additionally get a helpless standing since they cause weight to acquire. All carbs, nonetheless, are not made equivalent and are not normally swelling. Possibly you're putting on weight or not, depends on the structure and measure of the carbs you eat. Ensure you pick food sources wealthy in fiber and starch yet low in sugar. An exploration completed in 2015 shows that burning through 30 g of fiber daily will cause weight reduction, raise glucose levels, and bringing down circulatory strain. Having 30 gr of your

dietary fiber is definitely not a difficult task. They can be gotten by devouring an essential egg sandwich, Mediterranean chickpea grain, peanut butter with an apple, and dark pea's enchiladas with chicken.

- Sweet potatoes
- Beetroots
- Quinoa
- Oats
- Brown rice
- Bananas
- Mangoes
- Apples
- Kidney beans
- Pears

- Avocado

- Carrots

- Broccoli

- Brussels sprouts

- Almonds

- Chickpeas are remembered for the IF Carb food list.

For Fats

Fats may contribute 20% to 35% of your day-by-day calories, according to the 2015-2020 Dietary Guidelines for Americans. Soaked fat may not add over 10% of everyday calories, most remarkably. Given the structure, the lipids might be solid, deficient, or only in the middle. Trans fats, for instance, increment aggravation and decrease the "positive" cholesterol levels; notwithstanding, they raise "poor people" cholesterol levels. They're found in heated merchandise and seared food varieties. Immersed fats may increment cardiovascular danger. Well-qualified assessments on this differ, regardless. Eating these with some restraint is alright. Red meat, coconut oil, entire milk, and heated products have a high immersed fat substance. Sound fats contain monounsaturated in addition to polyunsaturated fats.

Such fats will bring down the danger of cardiovascular infection, bringing down blood pressure, even lower blood fat levels. Rich wellsprings of these fats are olive oil, canola oil, nut oil, safflower oil, sunflower oil, and soybean oils. The IF food list for fats ordinarily include:

- Avocados

- Nuts

- Cheese

- Whole eggs

- Dark chocolate

- Fatty fish

- Chia seeds

- Extra virgin olive oil (EVOO)

- Full-fat yogurt

For A Healthy Gut

A developing assortment of exploration proposes that the key to your ideal wellbeing is your gut. A great many microscopic organisms named the microbiota live in your stomach. Such microscopic organisms influence the soundness of your gut, your digestion even your psychological wellness. These can likewise be engaged with other persistent issues. Thus, you should care for those tiny bugs in your stomach, especially when you are fasting. The discontinuous fasting food list for a sound gut commonly includes:

- All veggies

- Fermented veggies

- Kefir

- Kimchi

- Kombucha

- Miso

- Sauerkraut

- Tempeh

To keep your gut sound, all food sources may likewise cause you to shed pounds by:

- Reducing the fat ingestion from the stomach.

- Increase discharge of ingested fat through stools.

- Decreasing food utilization.

For Hydration

According to the National Academies of Science, Engineering, and Medicine, the everyday fluid necessity for individuals is:

- For men, roughly 15.5 cups (3.7 liters).

- For ladies, about 11.5 cups (2.7 liters).

Liquids involve water and water-containing drinks. All through discontinuous fasting, remaining hydrated is vital for your wellbeing. Lack of hydration may lead to cerebral pains, extreme weariness, and dazedness. At the point when you are as yet managing these fasting results, lack of hydration could make them serious or much more limited.

The hydration rundown of irregular fasting food varieties incorporates:

- Coffee

- Sparkling water

- Tea or Black espresso

- Watermelon

- Strawberries

- Peaches

- Oranges

- Skim milk

- Lettuce

- Cucumber

- Celery

- Tomatoes

- Plain yogurt

Taking heaps of water can likewise help with getting in shape. An examination concentrate in 2016 notes that sufficient hydration will cause you to get thinner by:

- Reducing your hunger or utilization of food

- Rising fat consuming

Dinners excluded from the Intermittent Fasting list of food sources

- Processed food sources

- Refined grains

- Trans-fat

- Sweetened beverages

- Candy bars

- Processed meat

- Alcoholic beverages

Conclusion

Rapid weight loss hypnosis and deep sleep meditation are two of the most powerful tools for weight loss, and these new gentle methods are both easy to use while also being amazingly effective.

Rapid weight loss hypnosis works by focusing your mind on the feeling of being slim and healthy. When you're asleep at night, you'll be taken on a guided tour through a day in your life when you're at your ideal weight, so that even as you sleep, you can experience the pleasure of being slim. This is one way to improve your self-esteem, just like if you were living in a happy marriage or had fulfilled all your potential.

Another way to use rapid weight loss hypnosis is to focus on the feeling of being slim in every waking moment, while you're working, while you're eating, and as you walk down the street.

Do these things, and your body will begin to change. The truth is that if we pay constant attention to something, we can improve it. Become aware of what you don't like about your body and then focus on changing it, and soon your body will be different. Of course, this doesn't work overnight-mind power takes time to achieve results, but if you do this regularly for a week or two, then I guarantee it'll start working for you.

Deep sleep meditation is the easiest way to lose weight because it ensures that you'll get the right kind of rest, and that means you'll enjoy more energy during the day while also eating less food.

When you use deep sleep meditation, your mind will have far more clarity when it's time for breakfast, so you won't feel drowsy and tired. Rather than wolfing down a large amount of food before you go to work, all you have to do is imagine how wonderful it would feel if your body was slim and healthy, which will allow your body to reach its ideal weight in no time at all.

If you want the best results, then always remember that you have to be persistent if you're going to lose weight and keep it off. These great weight loss hypnosis techniques work even better when they're combined with other programs such as the fat-burning diet, so always choose quality over quantity when it comes to what you eat.

Your body will change as you lose weight, so be prepared for the unexpected and always have a positive attitude. This can only help you achieve success, so don't ever give up.

It's all about you, your health, and your happiness, and that's what matters.

Before using these tools to aid in your weight loss, you should consult your health care professional for an assessment of your weight loss goals and any associated risks. Your health care professional will be able to help you work out what is appropriate for you.

These weight loss hypnosis tools should not be used to replace a health care professional's recommendations.

BOOK 2 :

RAPID WEIGHT LOSS HYPNOSIS AND EMOTIONAL EATING

POWERFUL BRAIN TRAINING FOR MEN AND WOMEN TO CHANGE HABITS AND LOSE WEIGHT IN A SIMPLE AND FAST WAY WITH MOTIVATIONAL AFFIRMATIONS

Introduction

Despite the name, rapid weight loss hypnosis can't magically make you lose weight when you are eating foods that are making you unhealthy. In fact, it can be detrimental to your health if it causes you to ignore or abandon healthy habits in favor of quick fixes.

Rapid weight loss hypnosis and emotional eating look at how rapid weight loss hypnosis for emotional eaters has evolved over the last few decades and how some people may choose this form of therapy for reasons other than just for their physical weight loss goals. This article will show readers how this form of treatment can help with a range of emotional ills such as anxiety, depression, and eating disorders.

If you are one of those who are looking to lose weight and are doing it in order to impress others, you may not find the results you want. It works by helping your mind to make healthy eating habits more accessible and less likely to give in to constant temptation.

Instead of getting caught up in fad diets, you accept the fact that losing weight takes time and doesn't happen overnight. Your therapist can help you choose a diet plan that is tailored for your body type and lifestyle. The hypnosis helps reinforce positive messages about healthy eating and exercise so that you can be more successful at managing your weight long-term.

The success of a hypnotherapy program is dependent on your willingness to incorporate healthy lifestyle changes into your daily routine. It is important that you are honest with yourself and with your therapist about what is motivating you to lose weight.

Your therapist may assign you homework where he or she asks you to write down things that make you feel relieved, powerful, or inspired. This question will help guide the discussion when your sessions start up again so your therapist can focus on those emotions that are holding you back from achieving your weight loss goals. With hypnosis, this issue can finally be addressed and moved past so that you can make changes for yourself and start losing weight safely and effectively.

Why It Works

Through hypnosis, your therapist will help you find the root of emotional eating that is holding you back from losing weight. For example, you may have survived childhood neglect, abuse, or abandonment. Whatever it is, it's so deeply rooted in your subconscious mind that even if you got rid of the weight and returned to a happy childhood memory, the psychological issues that cause emotional eating would still be there.

A hypnotherapy program combats this issue by helping you understand how your post-traumatic stress disorder is affecting how you think and act in certain situations. Your therapist will help you to look at these situations in a more rational way instead of being overwhelmed. For example, your therapist might ask you to revisit a childhood memory and see it from a new perspective.

You will be coached by your therapist whether this idea applies to you or not. He or she will use emotional eating as the benchmark to show you how your day-to-day life is becoming more and more affected by your excessive emotional eating habits.

You will be guided into a deeper level of hypnosis where the old chains that bind you to overeat can be broken. Your therapist may also bring up some of your childhood abuse and neglect in order to help you connect the dots and see why your childhood experiences created these problems for you today.

Chapter 1 - Weight Loss Hypnosis

This hypnosis is going to be a way that will validate your weight loss goals. You will be able to recognize how relaxing and being peaceful throughout the weight loss process makes it easier to keep the pounds off. Keep an open mind with this, and remember to let thoughts flow naturally into your brain as if they were your own.

Hypnosis for Natural Weight Loss

You know how to relax your body. You are an expert at making sure that your limbs can hang freely without tension. We need to let our minds relax now.

Don't just let your body feel like jelly floating through the water. Let your mind be as malleable in this process too. With hypnosis, you have to let others into your head for just a moment. So allow your thoughts to flow freely and don't put any pressure on yourself to think a certain thing. Focus now on your breath.

Breathe in for five and out for five. Breathe in through your nose and out through your mouth. This is a way that's going to help make sure that you are focused on healthy living. Breathe in for one, two, three, four, and five, and out for five, four, three, two, and one.

Now we're going to do something a little different. Breathe in for five and then out for one long second. This time, we're only going to breathe in and out through your nose. Breathe in through your nose for one, two, three, four, and five, and out for one and a long and forceful breath.

You are slowly breathing in new air, and then you forcefully push it out as fast as you can. Breathe in for one, two, three, four, and five, and out for one with a quick snap. This way, you focus your breathing and make it easier for the air to flow in and out of your body.

You are going to want to snap your attention to nothing. You can look ahead of you now, but make sure that you get all of your sights out. On the count of three, you're going to snap your eyes closed and also breathe out at the same time.

So look around you and breathe in for one, two, three, four, and five. Now quickly shut your eyes and breathe out in one long breath. You can go back to regular breathing now but continue to focus on breathing in through your nose and out through your mouth. Try to do it in a pattern of five, but don't get too hung up on the strict structure. Instead, you'll want to focus on letting your thoughts come into your brain as if they were your own.

Keep your mind focused and breathe in. In front of you in your mind, only with your eyes closed, see the emergence of a spinning wheel. This wheel has nothing special about it. It is simply silver with rubber tires, and it is spinning fast. It is not attached to anything. It is simply a spinning wheel. It spins faster and faster and faster. Stare directly at the silver center. Notice how it continues to cycle through quickly.

Now that tire is turning into a circle of water. The water is flowing around as if it were a washing machine in which the water rotates in a circle.

The water is spinning and spinning. It is splashing against itself, but it is all still contained within this one simple silver circle. Continue to look at the center. There is nothing else around; everything is black. Notice this silver

224

spinning water. It goes over and over and over in a simple cycle in a simple loop. Focus on the center again as we count for your breathing. Breathe in for one, two, three, four, and five, and out for five, four, three, two, and one. Suddenly, on the count of three, this spinning cycle is going to snap into every corner of your mind. You are going to be engulfed in this spinning water.

One, two, and three. You are now in the water. You see around you that you are on a calm beach.

The water is not spinning anymore and is completely serene and clear. You walk towards the edge of the beach. You see it now that the water is slapping against the shore. This is the way that it was spinning around in circles in your mind.

No longer is it spinning now, and it is simply a normal ocean slapping against the beach. You can feel the water dripping off your skin, but the sun above you is already drying out. The sun is a vibrant yellow, and it casts a warm glow over your body. The sun kisses you at the top of your head and spreads down all the way to the tip of your toes. You look down at your feet and see that they're submerged in the sand. There is still water gently coming over and washing against your feet. You move your toes upwards, and they break through some of the sand, only for it to form quickly over them again. As the water smooths it out, you look ahead of you and breathe in again. You breathe in for one, two, three, four, and five, and out for five, four, three, two, and one, and notice all of these smells that come in with that. You breathe again for one, two, three, four, and five, and out for five, four, three, two, and one. You feel refreshed, energized, and free.

You are natural, pure, clean, and clear. You are part of this beach now with your feet stuck in the sand. You are like a tree with roots deep under the surface.

You decide now to sit down. Sink a little deeper into the sand. Water continues to emerge around you now like a warm blanket, all the way up to your hips. It keeps you feeling completely centered and pure on the now.

You look around you, to your right and left, and see that there are plenty of rocks. These, of course, don't hurt you. They just simply are part of the sand.

You dig your fingers into the sand, a little bit feeling the cold packed down underneath the initial warmth on the top of the surface. You dig out a rock and see that it is flat and smooth. You clear a little bit of this rock off using water as it passes over. You throw the rock quickly and sharply against the top of the water and watch as it jumps. It was a nice skipping rock that effortlessly glided across the top. You do this a few more times with other smooth and flat rocks that surround you. It is a reminder of how you can manipulate nature.

The water is getting higher and higher now, and you are chest-deep in the water. It is perfectly warm and calm, bringing plenty of waves back to the surface. You want to feel the sun on your skin again now, so you decide to stand up.

You walk across the sand, now in the dry area. Sand begins to stick to your legs, but still, it is nice and warm. You walk across, feeling your feet sink deep in. Each new step you take, the bottom of your foot is hot from the surface of the sand. It adjusts quickly as it sinks down, and you feel a sensation over and over again as you continue to walk. You see ahead of you that there is what looks to be a sandcastle. As you get closer and closer, you see that there is no castle at all. It is simply a wall that somebody has built with the sand. You decide to walk all the way through this wall now.

No longer is there something that is going to block off part of the beach. It was simply made of sand, so it was easy for you to destroy with your feet and legs only. As you walk through this section, you recognize that this is a representation of the walls that you have built around yourself. You will no longer let yourself be afraid of the things that you want. You can't just be comfortable with the situation you're in anymore. Being comfortable does not always mean being happy. You want to be able to feel completely fresh and pure. You're not attached to the things that you used to be or the person that used to keep your mind stuck in the same situations over and over again.

You sit in the middle of the now-destroyed wall and look out on the beach again. The sun continues to send warm feelings all across your skin.

You breathe in deeply, feeling this ocean air fill your body once again. These oceans are responsible for so much. They are the life force that keeps everybody moving. We take fish from the ocean, and it helps us travel and carry things across waters. You breathe. All of this is a reminder of the incredible world that you're a part of.

While your problems and issues are valid, this is also a reminder of how small some things that seem like such big deals to us really are in the grand scheme of things. There is a great and powerful force that exists just within the world alone.

You are an important part of this, and it is a reminder of the incredible and powerful person that you are. The sun is setting, so you decide to go for one last and final dip before you don't have the chance anymore. You don't want to swim in the dark, so you decide to wade in a little bit and get your last dose of ocean water right now.

You walk in, and the water is all the way up to your hip. You can look down and see the ocean floor because the water is so clear. You don't really see any fish, but you can see the old shells leftover by different crabs or other ocean critters.

You walk a little bit further, and now the water is up to your chest. The waves are so gentle you barely feel them. It's almost as if you were in a deep and warm bath because the water is so relaxing.

You decide to lift your legs up now. Floating on top of the water, you simply move around, letting the waves take you where you need to go. If you go out too far from the shore or off to the side too much, you can gently guide yourself back to where you want to be with a simple arm or leg movement. You are simply free in the water, almost as if you're flying through the sky.

There is no gravity at this moment. You breathe in and out, in and out. The water is surrounding you now. A few droplets will get on your face here and there as the water continues to splash around you, but nothing too extreme. You close your eyes for just a moment, letting the water wash over your face.

You are clean, pure, natural, and energized at this moment. Breathe in for five and out for five. Breathe in for five and out for five. Everything around you is turning black. Darkness begins to consume you once again, and you realize you are now back in your bed on the couch, ready to start a new life. You feel yourself slowly falling into your bed, and you are waking up.

The person this dream was about is no longer there, and you start to open your eyes.

The bedroom is overwhelmingly bright with a white-yellow glow. The second you open your eyes, the brightness seems to calm down slowly, as if it were just that—a dream.

You feel refreshed, pure, free, and clear now after having this dream. You begin to wonder what else you can do with this technique or practice because it is something that still gives you great inspiration even weeks later. The technique above for lucid dreaming has been used at least 200 times or more by some people reading my blog post.

I want to give you the full list of feedback that I've received on this blog post.

1.   At the start, I wasn't too sure about creating a new technique that I never tested out before. But if you read my blog, then you will know that this technique has been very useful for me and my clients.

2.   It has changed my life! Before, I had completely lost control of my life and was living in a total mess! Now, after applying this technique to lucid dreaming, life has completely transformed.

3.   I've read about it and tried it out. It worked for me. The most important thing is to understand the idea behind it and then have the right mindset, intention, and belief in your own self to go through with the process of lucid dreaming.

4.   When I first read about this, I was confused with everything in my head. But, when I started trying it, I kept on doing it every day and now I

am able to control my dreams whenever I want to without an alarm clock or medication! Thanks, Siddharth.

5.   This is a very useful technique that can be used for many purposes. I have used it to experience different situations and emotions. It gives a very quick and effective result.

6.   This technique is liberating in nature since it is directly facilitating you to control your dreams rather than relying on external sources like wishful thinking or luck. The best part is that once you have gained confidence, it can be used many times in your life in different ways.

7.   I have tried this process before but I could not do it properly back then until I read your blog post about how to do it and apply the technique properly to achieve lucid dreaming successfully!

8.   Lucid dreaming is just a dream, but this method of lucid dreaming control gives you much more control over it. If you are ever going to get to the point where you can achieve full control of your dreams, then you must definitely try this technique. This technique and its purpose can help a lot many people with their daily lives and even with their health as well.

9.   I am not sure if practicing this is useful or not, but I feel like I need to use some techniques that are effective than just sitting in some activity that doesn't actually motivate me into doing anything at all. It is very feasible that the routine would be repetitive and useless in the long run. I would also want to explore the possibility at a later time when I have more time.

10.   This technique is very useful for lucid dreaming if you believe in yourself and want to achieve it. Keep on practicing, and you will eventually

see great results that will motivate you even more into doing things that are related to lucid dreams.

11.   It is a very simple practice, but it can be effective for many reasons as long as you know what your intentions are behind lucid dreaming. If you plan on using this technique to only achieve something like going back in time or any sort of manipulations of things in the real world then expect failure most of the time as it is just a dream after all!

Chapter 2 - Meditation Exercise for Rapid Weight Loss Hypnosis

Meditation Exercise 1—Release of Bad Habits

Sit comfortably. Relax your muscles, close your eyes. Breathe in and breathe out. Do not cross your feet because this will lock you away from the desired experience. Hold your hands together to connect your logical brain hemisphere with your instinct.

Concentrate on your back now and notice how you feel in the bed or chair you are sitting in. Take a deep breath and let your stress leave your body. Now focus on your neck. Observe how your neck is joined to your shoulders.

Lift your shoulders slowly. Breathe in slowly and release it. Feel how your shoulders loosen. Lift your shoulders again a little bit then let them relax. Observe how your neck muscles are tensing and how much pressure it has.

Breathe in and breathe out slowly. Release the pressure in your neck and notice how the stress is leaving your body. Repeat the whole exercise from the beginning. Observe your back. Notice all the stress and let it go with a profound breath. Focus on your shoulders and neck again. Lift up your shoulders and hold it for some moments, then release your shoulders again and let all the stress go away. Sense how the stress is going away. Now, focus your attention on your back. Feel how comfortable it is. Focus on your whole body. While breathing in, let relaxation come, and while you are breathing out, let frustration leave your body. Notice how much you are relaxed.

Concentrate on your inner self. Breathe slowly in and release it. Calm your mind. Observe your thoughts. Don't go with them because your aim is to observe them and not to be involved. It's time to let go of your overweight self that you are not feeling good about. It's like your body is wearing a bigger, heavier top at this point in your life. Imagine stepping out of it and laying it on an imaginary chair facing you. Now tell yourself to let go of.

These old, established eating and behavioral patterns. Imagine that all your old, fixed patterns and all the obstacles that prevent you from achieving your desired weight are exiting your body, soul, and spirit with each breath. Know that your soul is perfect as it is, and all you want is for everything that pulls away to leave. With every breath, let your old beliefs go, as you are creating more and more space for something new. After spending a few minutes with this, imagine that every time you breathe in, you are inhaling prana, the life energy of the universe shining in gold. In this life force, you will find everything you need and desire: a healthy, muscular body, a self that loves itself in all circumstances, a hand that puts enough nutritious food on the table, a strong voice to say no to sabotaging your diet, a head that can say no to those who are trying to distract you from your ideas and goals. With each breath, you absorb these positive images and emotions.

See in front of you exactly what your life would be like if you got everything you wanted. Release your old self and start becoming your new self.

Gradually restore your breathing to regular breathing. Feel the solid ground beneath you, open your eyes, and return to your everyday state of consciousness.

Meditation Exercise 2—Forgiving Yourself

Imagine a staircase in front of you! Descend it, counting down from ten to one. You reached and found a door at the bottom of the stairs. Open the door. There is a meadow in front of us. Let's see if it has grass, if so: Does it have flowers? What color? If there are bushes or trees, describe what you see in the distance.

Find the path covered with white stones and start walking on it. Feel the power of the Earth flowing through your soles, the breeze stroking your skin, the warmth of the sun radiating toward you. Feel the harmony of the elements and your state of well-being.

From the left side, you hear the rattle of the stream. Walk down to the shore. This water of life comes from the throne of God. Take it with your palms and drink three sips and notice how it tastes. If you want, you can wash in it. Keep walking. Feel the power of the Earth flowing through your soles, the breeze stroking your skin, the warmth of the sun radiating toward you.

Feel the harmony of the elements and your state of well-being. In the distance, you see an ancient tree with many branches. This is the Tree of Life.

Take a leaf from it, chew it, and note its taste. You have arrived at the Lake of Conscience. No one in this lake sinks. Rest on the water and think that all the emotions and thoughts you no longer need (anger, fear, horror,

235

hopelessness, pain, sorrow, anxiety, annoyance, self-blame, superiority, self-pity, and guilt) pass through your skin and you purify them by the magical power of water. And you see that the water around you is full of gray and black globules that are slowly recovering the turquoise-green color of the water.

You feel the power of the water, the power of the Earth, the breeze of your skin, the radiance of the sun warming you, the harmony of the elements, the feeling of well-being.

You ask your magical horse to come for you. You love your horse; you pamper it and let it caress you too. You bounce on its back and head to God's Grad. In the air, you fly together, become one being. You have arrived.

Ask your horse to wait. You grow wings, and you fly toward the Trinity. You bow your head and apologize for all the sins you have committed against your body. You apologize for all the sins you have committed against your soul. You apologize for all the sins you committed against your spirit. You wait for the angels to give you the gifts that help you. If you can't see yourself receive one, it means you don't need one yet. If you did, open it and look inside.

Give thanks that you could be here. Get back on your horse and fly back to the meadow. Find the white gravel path and head back down to the door to your stairs. Look at the grass in the meadow. Notice if there are any flowers.

If so, describe the colors, any bush or tree, and whatever you see in the distance. You arrive at the door, open it, and head up the stairs. Count from one to ten. You are back, move your fingers slowly, open your eyes.

Meditation Exercise 3—Rapid Weight Loss

See yourself in every detail. Describe your hair, the color of your clothes, your eyes. See your face, your nose, your mouth. Set aside this image for a moment. Now imagine yourself as you would like to be in the future. Imagine that your new self-approaching your present self and pampers it. See that your new self-embracing your present self. Feel the love that is spread in the air. Now see that your present self leaves the scene and your new self takes its place.

See and feel how happy and satisfied you are. You believe that you can become this beautiful new self. You breathe in this image and place it in your soul. This image will always be with you and flow through your whole body.

You want to be this new self. You can be this new self. This is your vision for life, and you have found love.

Meditation Exercise 4—Inner Peace

First, visualize the things that make you feel safe and happy. See everything in detail. See the colors of the objects and what they are made of, whether they are new or old. Listen to all the sounds around you: cars, birds chirping, a fountain in someone's yard, people talking on their cell phones as they walk down the street. Listen to all these sounds and focus on how peaceful it is here right now and now only.

Then imagine your heart. See its color and feel the warmth and love in your heart. After this, your mind will naturally start to relax and slow down. You will feel calm. This is the time when you sleep!

You want to be this new self. You can be this new self. This is your vision for life, and you have found love.

The meditation exercise guides the practitioner from identifying his or her fears to setting a new course for life based on acceptance of the present moment and an appreciation for life's beauty along with acceptance of hardships and challenges that make human existence different from pleasure-seeking animals that act without thought or purposeful action. The exercises also offer a sense of peace and well-being in the consciousness of the practitioner. The main goal of the four meditations is to achieve a state of mind that allows the practitioner to set goals for future success, reach them despite obstacles, keep away from bad habits, block negative thoughts and feelings, and achieve inner peace.

Chapter 3 - Hypnotherapy for Weight Loss. Does It Work?

Hypnosis might be more viable than diet and exercise alone for individuals hoping to get thinner. The thought is that the brain can be affected to change propensities like indulging. Be that as it may, precisely how powerful it might be is still easy to refute.

The specialists inferred that while this extra misfortune wasn't noteworthy, hypnosis therapy justified more exploration as a treatment for corpulence.

A Trusted Source analysis that included hypnotherapy, explicitly intellectual conduct treatment (CBT), for weight reduction, indicated that it brought about a small decrease in body weight contrasted and the fake treatment gathering.

Specialists reasoned that while hypnotherapy may upgrade weight reduction, there isn't sufficient examination for it to be persuasive.

What Is in Store from Hypnotherapy?

During hypnotherapy, your specialist will probably start your meeting by clarifying how hypnosis functions. At that point, they will go over your objectives. From that point, your specialist may start talking in a calming, delicate voice to assist you with unwinding and to set up a sentiment of security.

Certain words or the redundancy of specific expressions may help with this stage. Your specialist may likewise assist you with envisioning yourself arriving at objectives through sharing clear mental symbolism.

To close the meeting, your advisor will help take you out of hypnosis and back to your beginning state. The length of the hypnosis meeting and the number of complete sessions you may need will rely upon your objectives.

Is Weight Reduction Hypnosis Compelling?

Weight reduction hypnosis may assist you with shedding an additional couple of pounds when it's a piece of a weight-reduction plan that incorporates diet, exercise, and guiding. In any case, it's difficult to state because there isn't sufficiently strong logical proof about weight reduction hypnosis alone.

Hypnosis is a condition of internal ingestion and fixation, such as being in a daze. Hypnosis is typically finishing with the assistance of a subliminal specialist utilizing verbal redundancy and mental pictures.

At the point when you're under hypnosis, your consideration is profoundly engaged, and you're more receptive to recommendations, including conduct changes that can assist you with getting in shape.

Be that as it may, an ongoing report, which just demonstrated direct weight reduction results, found that patients accepting hypnosis had lower paces of irritation, better satiety, and better personal satisfaction. These may be components whereby hypnosis could impact weight. Further investigations expect to comprehend completely the possible job of hypnosis in the field of executives.

Weight reduction usually is best accomplished with diet and exercise. If you've attempted an eating regimen and practice, however, are as yet battling to meet your weight reduction objective, converse with your human services supplier about different alternatives or ways of life changes that you can make.

All That You Need to Know About Using Hypnosis for Weight Loss

You're likely suspicious. That is because Hollywood has given us a quite specific, and wrong, picture of what a trance specialist does and can do. "You won't transform into a zombie or cackle like a chicken," says Valorie Wells, Ph.D., a clinical hypnosis expert in Kansas City, MO. Hypnotherapy is extraordinarily only you revealing to yourself however you wish you to be, despite whether it's to rest higher, to induce agent, to drive on a drive at soap throttle between 2 trucks.

And keeping in mind that examination is scant, what we do have says hypnosis works shockingly well. Early investigations found that individuals who utilized hypnosis lost more than twice as much weight as the individuals who ate less without the treatment. An examination in the International Journal of Clinical and Experimental Hypnosis discovered ladies who experienced Hypno behavioral therapy shed pounds, improved their dietary patterns, and improved their self-perception. In the interim, a meta-examination by British scientists found hypnosis could help manage the arrival of peptides that control how eager and full you feel.

Who Should Try It?

It is vital because the core of why hypnosis works is because it instructs you to have more determination. "Individuals who see me for weight reduction, food have assumed an inappropriate position in their brain," Wells clarifies.

The objective of hypnotherapy is to revamp this affiliation. "We need to re-incorporate the possibility that food is fuel."

How It Works

Wells includes that nothing she does is scrip and, other than the message that food is fuel, the entrancing recommendations are tweaking dependent on this underlying discussion.

After the talk, you move into the hypnosis meeting, which keeps going around 20 to 25 minutes. "What I'm doing is helping this individual equalization the voices in their mind," Wells clarifies.

We as a whole have a stable inner mind—the gut response that keeps you out of threat or aides great choices that internal voice is that the one that shields North American country from acting solely on feeling. "Throughout hypnosis, everything I am doing is cranking the quantity informed that inward intelligence and down on the emotional half," she clarifies.

What does that stable like it? Wells says a case of a mesmerizing recommendation may be: "You will go after new organic product. You will perceive desserts are excessively overwhelming for you and that new natural product will cause you to feel fulfilled and supported."

What Is Hypnosis and What Is It for?

Spellbinding—or hypnotherapy—utilizes guided unwinding, serious fixation, and centered regard to accomplishing an elevated condition of mindfulness that is once in a while called a daze. The individual's consideration is so engaged while in this express anything going on around the individual is briefly shut out or overlooked. Spellbinding viewed as 'a waking condition of mindfulness, (or cognizance), in which an individual's consideration is confined from their quick condition and consumed by inward encounters, for example, emotions, comprehension, and imagery.'

Hypnotic enlistment includes the centering of consideration and creative inclusion to where the envisioned feels genuine. By the utilization and acknowledgment of proposals, the clinician and patient build a mesmerizing reality. Regular 'daze' states are a piece of our everyday human experience, for example, losing all sense of direction in a decent book, driving down a comfortable stretch of street with no conscious memory, when in petition or reflection, or when undertaking a dreary or an innovative action. Our cognizant familiarity with our environmental factors versus inward mindfulness is on a continuum, so that, when in these states, one's center is overwhelmingly inside, yet one doesn't lose all external mindfulness.

Hypnosis views as a thoughtful state, which one can figure out how to get to intentionally and purposely, for a therapeutic reason. Recommendations are then given either verbally or utilizing symbolism, coordinated at the ideal result. It may be to mollify nervousness by getting to serenity and unwinding, help oversee reactions of meds, or assist ease with tormenting or different indications. Contingent upon the recommendations given, spellbinding is typically a loosening up understanding, which can be exceptionally helpful with a patient who is tense or restless. Be that as it may, the fundamental helpfulness of the fascinating state is the expanded viability of recommendation and access to mind/body connections or oblivious preparation. Entrancing cannot exclusively use to lessen enthusiastic trouble, yet additionally may directly affect the patient's understanding of pain.

Hypnosis is a psychological state of exceptionally engaged fixation, lessened fringe mindfulness, and uplifted suggestibility. There are various procedures that specialists utilize for actuating such a state. Exploiting the intensity of proposal, hypnosis is regularly used to help individuals unwind, to lessen the vibe of agony, or to encourage some ideal social change. Specialists achieve hypnosis (likewise alluded to as hypnotherapy or hypnotic recommendation) with the assistance of mental symbolism and the mitigation of verbal redundancy that slides the patient into a dazed state. When loose, patients' psyches are more open to groundbreaking messages. Not every person is similarly hypnotizable. Utilizing mind imaging strategies, specialists have discovered contrasts in examples of cerebrum availability between the individuals who react to hypnotic acceptance and the individuals who don't. The differentiation appears in the hypnotizable as elevated co-enactment between the chief control place in the prefrontal cortex and another piece of the prefrontal cortex that hails the significance, or notability of occasions.

The Uses of Hypnosis

As opposed to mainstream thinking, people remain alert during hypnosis and, for the most part, review their encounters. Under the direction of a prepared social insurance proficient, hypnosis can be utilized to ease torment, treat immune system ailment, battle fears, and end unfortunate

244

propensities, for example, smoking and indulging. Hypnosis can likewise assist individuals with adapting to negative passionate states, similar to stress and uneasiness, just as torment, exhaustion, sleep deprivation, temperament issues, and the sky is the limit from there.

What method would hypnosis be able to support you? Hypnosis has been utilized rather than sedatives to diminish torment and uneasiness when medical procedures. It additionally appears to help to mend from numerous conditions, including epilepsy, neuralgia, ailment, and skin conditions. The physiological and neurological changes that happen under hypnosis are like oneself recuperating misleading impact—an instance of the brain over the issue.

What Makes Somebody Simple to Mesmerize?

As opposed to generalizations, hypnosis works best when an individual is a willing member. A few people are more open to hypnotic proposals than others. Specialists call this attribute "hypnotizability" and perceive that it can shift significantly among people. Indeed, even individuals with significant levels of hypnotizability may require numerous hypnosis meetings to see improvement.

Two hypnosis are not treatments. However, it very well may be a device that encourages the conveyance of treatment similarly as a needle conveys drugs. Entrancing doesn't make the incomprehensible conceivable; however, it can assist patients with accepting and experience what may be workable for them to accomplish. Alluring states have been utilized for mending since humankind has existed. Still, since spellbinding can be abused for alleged diversion and has been depicted in the media as something puzzling and supernatural, as far as anyone knows out of the mesmerizing subject's control, it has been seen with doubt and distrust by numerous well-being experts. Be that as it may, late advances in neuroscience have empowered us to start to comprehend what may be occurring when somebody enters a mesmerizing state, three and proof is working for the utilization of fascinating as a valuable instrument to support patients, and well-being experts deal with an assortment of conditions, particularly nervousness and agony. As clinicians, we realize that just realizing something doesn't interpret having the option to control feelings, for example, dread and uneasiness. A straightforward 'model' that uses to assist patients with understanding this is a severe normal reaction is that of right/left mind, which can likewise correspond with cognizant/oblivious and scholarly/passionate handling. From the graph, it tends to see that to convey successfully the two kinds of our handling; we need more than words; we have to utilize words that inspire symbolism. It is nothing unexpected, in this way, that all the best educators use representation, anecdote, and story to pass on their lessons.

Conclusion

Wells says, "People with obesity problems and strong weight issues will figure out things that will go into the way of their progress." The objective is to get you unstuck. We are not going to turn you into a zombie or either cackle like a chicken. Wells says.

Rather, we're working with the idea that you have a voice in your mind that is sending out messages like, "You must eat less!" and, "You should be careful about what you eat because it makes you fat," she clarifies.

Wells says that the quality of the hypnotic state really changes from individual to individual. "Hypnosis is a more intense circumstance than resting. One individual may observe it as a night of light sleep. Another experiences more intense hypnosis—whether it's to put forth a greater amount of power, eat less or unwind."

"My goal is for clientele to feel more empowered and in charge of their own choices and destinies," she explains.

Chapter 4 - Getting Started with Weight Loss Hypnosis

Are you ready to kick start your weight loss journey? There are several options to start from. It would be great to visit a professional hypnotherapist for a physical session or fix a virtual conference with a hypnotherapist.

Another alternative is the recorded hypnosis or self-hypnosis. All the hypnosis methods have shown promising results for weight loss.

One-on-one hypnosis-A hypnotherapist can help you recognize the unconscious limitations that hold you in bond. Additionally, in those sessions, a hypnotherapist sees you solving the limitations.

These are performed in workplaces or by video conferencing instead.

Guided Hypnosis

A guided record of hypnosis can help you get started quickly and learn the mechanisms of hypnosis at your home or on the go.

More importantly, these are records of certified hypnotherapists who walk you through induction and then give positive suggestions through the recording.

Self-hypnosis; participating in self-hypnosis, individuals assume hypnotherapist accountability, allowing them to use a memorized script to trick them into hypnosis and then give constructive suggestions. Get lost in every habit and reach your targets for weight loss.

Close your eyes; watch your food cravings go off, picture a day eating exactly what's best for you. Eventually, imagine hypnosis helping you lose weight because the news is; it does. Here are ten hypnotic suggestions to try immediately.

Many people have not come to know and recognize that adding trance to your weight loss scheme can help you lose more weight and keep it farther off.

Hypnosis precedes calorie counting by a few centuries, but the long-age strategies have not been considered, not completely accepting it as an efficient weight-loss strategy. There has been scant scientific evidence recently to support the legitimate resolutions of respected hypnotherapists,

Even after the convincing evaluations of 18 hypnotic research studies in the mid-nineties revealed that psychotherapy clients who learned self-hypnosis lost twice as much weight as those who didn't. Thus, hypnotherapy has been a well-kept mystery of weight loss.

Until you or someone you know has been happily forced by hypnosis to buy a new, smaller wardrobe, it can be quite difficult to be convinced that this mind-over technique could help you get a handle on eating.

You Believe What You See

So see for yourself. You don't necessarily need to be in trance to get some of the priceless lessons about weight loss that hypnosis has to teach. The ten mini-ideas that follow contain some of the diet-altering suggestions that my patients receive in the team and individual hypnotherapy for weight management.

1.   **The answer is within.** Hypnotherapists think that you are already embedded in everything you need to succeed. You do not even need another crash diet or a recent appetite suppressant. Slimming is about reminding yourself of your natural skills, just like when you're riding a bike. You may not remember how scary you were initially trying to ride, but you continued to rehearse until you could ride automatically, without effort or deep thinking. Weight loss can look beyond you equally, but the truth is, it's about finding a balance.

2.   **You see what you believe.** People seem to be getting what they think they can achieve. That applies to hypnosis, too. Those tricked into thinking that they could be hypnotized (for example, according to the hypnotist's suggestion, they should see how blue flips the switch of a hidden blue light bulb) displayed enhanced hypnotic sensitivity. The expectation that help will be given is crucial. It's my suggestion that you expect to work out your weight loss plan.

3.   **Positive intensifies.** Negative or opposing ideas such as "potato chips would sicken you" have been working for a while, but if you need a permanent improvement, you would have been better you think positive. A hypnotherapy team developed the most common hypnotic suggestion: "excessive food is dangerous for my body. I need my body to live. It is my duty to respect and protect my body." I encourage customers to put buoyant mantras down. A mother of fifty, who lost more than fifty pounds, repeats daily; unnecessary food is a burden on my body. I'm going to shed what I don't want.

251

4.   **If you can visualize it, it will come.** Just like we've got athletes primed for competition, envisaging victory gets you prepared for a victorious reality. Envisaging a day of healthy eating helps you visualize the steps needed to become that healthy eater. Too hard to grasp? Look out for an old picture of yourself at a soothing and beautiful weight and remember what you did differently, then imagine bringing those routines back to function or imagine getting a piece of advice from a future older, wiser self after reaching her desired weight.

5.   **Send in the abnormal food flying appetite.** Hypnotherapists make repeated use of the power of symbolic imagery, inviting subjects to put their food cravings on soft white clouds or balloons in hot air, and send them up and away. A hypnotist is aware that counter symbols are drawing you back. Engage the mind to search pages of images until one emerges as a sign of casting out cravings.

6.   **Double strategies are better than a single one.** The combination that ascertains reaching the ideal target when it comes to holding off weight is hypnosis and cognitive-behavioral therapy, which aims to change negative thoughts and behaviors. Customers with the knowledge of the two have been told to lose twice as much weight without falling into the loss of some by the dieter, to regain more trap. If you've ever kept a food note, you've already tried CBT. They keep records of goes by their lips for a week or two before clients study hypnosis. Increasing awareness, as any skilled hypnotherapist knows, is a vital step towards continuous progress.

7.   **Modify and modify.** Milton Erickson, MD, a recent initiator of hypnosis, stressed the importance of harnessing existing patterns. To change the lose-recovery, lose-recovery pattern of a client, Erickson

suggested that she must gain weight first and then lose it—a difficult way nowadays. Modify the cravings for peak calories. Instead of an ice cream tip, not consider a cup of frozen yogurt?

8. **It is the survival of the fattest.** No suggestion is sufficiently potent to subdue the survival instinct. Although we would like to believe that it is survival for the fittest, we're all conditioned for the survival of the fattest in the case of famine. A private nutritional coach wanted me to recommend a way out of her gummy bear habit; I tried to illustrate that her body felt that her life depended on the chewy sweets and wouldn't give up on them until she got enough calories from the nutritious foods. No, she has persisted; what she needed was a suggestion. That she dropped out was no surprise.

9. **You become perfect in whatever you practice.** A Pilate class doesn't result in washboard abs, and only one hypnotic session won't modify your diet. Still, the quiet constant repetition of a positive suggestion of up to fifteen to twenty minutes a day will improve your eating, usually when paired with soft, natural breaths, the basis of any behavioral change scheme.

10. **Congratulations—this is a relapse.** I congratulate clients when they see themselves contradicting their healthiest goals, and overindulging. Hypnosis addresses a relapse as an avenue, not a travesty. If you can learn from a true or potential relapse—why it happened, how to treat it differently—you'll be better prepared for the inevitable temptations of life. You can be more compassionate with yourself, a state that precedes change.

12.   **It is not for everyone.** This is true: Hypnosis doesn't work for everyone, as talking and listening do not work for everyone. Yet two million people in the United States use hypnotic methods daily to quit smoking, lose weight, and stop their compulsive eating habits. I have said this to students over the years: A trained hypnotist cannot hypnotize them against their will under any circumstance—it's an artifact of stage shows where a hypnotist asks you to do something silly and embarrassing, like take off your clothes or kiss someone on stage. But the reason I stress that an individual must be willing to be hypnotized is due to the fact that some people resist. It is their resistance that keeps them from being hypnotized.

Chapter 5 - The Human Mind

The weight reduction industry is basic information that just an eating routine or a health improvement plan doesn't guarantee enduring weight reduction results. You will perpetually recuperate all weight if you don't accept that you are thin and solid for life in your oblivious brain. This is one territory that is inadequate in most weight decrease programs. There is, nonetheless, an approach to finish this lost connection. We like to consider our brains and bodies as being various elements; however, both are connected more intently than we might suspect.

You will realize this is substantial on the off chance that you have at any point perused of individuals getting minor medical procedures affected by only spellbinding. The more significant part of us is happy to have sedatives under these conditions. However, it shows precisely how solid the psyche can be!

Could the Mind Affect the Body's Well-being?

Indeed, it does—which is why it delivers profits to zero in effectively utilizing the brain's force. We as a whole can think of either particular or negative contemplations all day long. If we need to believe adversely, it can significantly affect our true prosperity.

For example, you can be the individual who gets discouraged and anxious significantly quicker. If anything ends up causing you to feel like this, it can influence how your body reacts to the circumstance; nonetheless. You can improve.

If you end up in a line, for instance, and for the most part, begin feeling focused at the measure of time you are squandering, change your reasoning. Take some full breaths and consider beneficial things. Likewise, you can utilize the time valuably and productively, perhaps by conversing with the individual close to you. The contention is that you ought to be idealistic in the present circumstance.

You decide to run out of the store. You needed to pause or feel fulfilled because you had a decent talk with somebody. Deal with the connection between psyche and body. Attempt presently to see what your feelings mean for the actual way you feel.

Stress can impact us from various perspectives. Long-haul pressure does minimal excellent to anybody; on the off chance that you realize that you are inclined to high pressure, attempt to ease it by utilizing your brain's solidarity.

Start with the mind and follow the rest. This is similarly evident when you start another course or dispatch another business with weight reduction. The thought is that you should initially convince your oblivious brain that you need to shed pounds and that you are a lean and adjusted individual.

It would be best to take care of these ideas in your subliminal self so your psyche can manage you to the possible choices that will understand these ideas.

Logical proof recommends that our ability to get criticism is subject to a particular perspective, a sort of altered perspective. This perspective is a takeoff from typical awareness, which fundamentally works under the Beta brainwave. At the point when it works, the mind produces electrochemical releases.

Nonetheless, there are diverse element levels. You are in beta while you work at your "alert" daytime stage—converse with companions, address somebody, read, tackle a compound condition, or compose an article. Beta waves range in recurrence from 15 to 40 cycles each second. This is the typical brainwave recurrence during the day. When you sit back after science issues have been addressed, you are in an Alpha state. When you sit on the train, you are in the Alpha state, and you watch the view streaming while your contemplations go on their excursion. It additionally puts you in this state to ask or contemplate.

Alpha cerebrum waves are slower yet more significant. Its recurrence shifts from 9–14 cycles each second. At the point when you are agreeable in this state, you feel quiet and safe. You have muscles and are available to ideas. The couple of moments you spend unwinding before nodding off are the Alpha state. It's ideal to re-program yourself to the Alpha state. 85% of all clinical issues (counting gorging and weight issues) incorporate uncertain body agony and stress. Getting to Alpha would assist you with upsetting this unsteady pressure and make your eating regimen more gradual. Additionally, when you consider Alpha, you can, without much of a stretch, reinvent yourself. Start by setting aside the effort to unwind.

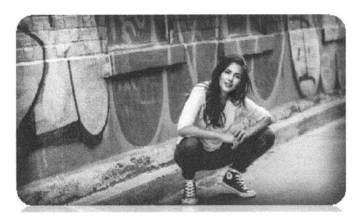

A reflective, tranquil day is 20–30 minutes in length enough. Assemble a profound breathing schedule that zeros in your psyche on a sentence, sound, or mantra. The meaning of the sound or word isn't just about as basic as it brings out in you. At the point when your body pressure has released, feed your brain with positive pictures.

Envision the ideal weight—think of your slim, lean body and shapely legs. Envision for yourself a healthy and dynamic life. Make it a customary practice for your optimal self in this empowering representation until you can genuinely consider yourself lean, solid, and excellent. Next time you want to wolf in a chocolate cake, transforming your brain into a thin body and thin legs.

It was tough for me to figure I should return to estimate 4 when I got an additional load during menopause. Presently the hormonal movements make it unthinkable for me to be what I was in my twenties. I reviewed then that I utilized a similar contention as I had made during my pregnancy: "Moms should put on weight."

We appear to rely upon commonly acknowledged speculations to decide. Do you realize that your body can be cut as you need? You're 99% water and quantum space, and when you see it, the body isn't tossed into stone or tissue.

Moreover, the visual cortex at the rear of the skull makes what you find in your cerebrum from an organization of substance and electric charges. Your visual cortex design differs from the example that another person or I create. You don't see anything out there. On the off chance that you visit, here you make things (your brain).

Presently we are liberated by that physiological truth - and we realize that we can make what we need now, and we can do it in any case if it's not what we need!!!

How Would We Be Able to Respond?

1.   Protein makes a thin weight, giving the body energetic strength by eating low-fat protein (not all that much creature protein joined with fat and calories).

2.   We can start an exercise like tennis, skating, strolling.

3.   We should cherish solid, nutritious food and eat great food.

4.   We should avoid the individuals who are attempting to eradicate our resolve.

We are liable for who we will be. Nothing attaches us to intrigue except for our feeling of requirement! Reflection is a decent start, yet you can't do it in a line!

A few groups are more romantic than others; however, luckily, you will turn out to be surer when attempting to get things going. A solid method to begin the connection between psyche and body is to practice consistently.

Most importantly, a short stroll in the first part of the day awakens your brain; it cautions you totally and helps your body feel great chemicals. It likewise has excellent actual outcomes and causes you to feel more idealistic as the day advances.

Preparing the Mind for Positive Output

Brain science gave us a scope of assets in programming social changes and thought enhancements to improve a person's state of mind or help this individual better face everyday certainties.

Different methodologies, like contemplation, spellbinding, and rest programming, are clinically concentrated. Nonetheless, mind activities and tests with mental boosts empower the individuals who need to prepare their brains themselves and give inconspicuous preparation to improve the psyche's force. The brain has effectively been pre-customized from our past encounters and learning. Our memories energize the work and give the premise of reference and differentiation of things that are found.

Any work to adjust what is now the main priority, change recently imagined thoughts, and guarantee that the psyche can endure more than it has done in the past requires a clear difference in mentality in an individual. Each individual decides how they decipher what they see and see and what they envision.

It is as yet our acumen that assembles all the information our cerebrum has gone through. Anyway incredible the mind is, one should note that it is still just a human device, and toward the day's end, it is our finished selves that will proceed to create and advance.

It is challenging to program mind insights, especially for skeptics and pragmatists. Rather than a liquid progression of cerebrum capacities, negative contemplations block ideal thoughts put away in our memory banks, giving our psyches a more challenging opportunity to sift through which ecological components are resources for accomplishing our charming state.

Likewise, it is critical to keep an uplifting mentality, as this will assist us with choosing what we need and which things move.

This ideological perspective is helped all the more effectively by adding each experience equivalent to our greatness or ideal standard. If we have a particular circumstance and can accomplish it with our minds' force, we will have a more substantial likelihood of making similar progress later.

This is all because of the adjusted perspective we currently have due to the past presentation. Without a doubt, the product idea can do a great deal since it clears the brain and makes it simpler to consider the ideal.

We should be in complete control of programming mind arrangements, thoughts, and recollections for execution. We need to understand what we need and how we need it to be done, and we should figure out how to think, dream and imagine it ourselves and our psyches, and we'll know soon that we live it as of now.

Chapter 6 - Magic Calorie Melt & Fat Burning

Excited much? You should be! Today is a big day. Today you begin your journey to permanent weight loss success and a brand new you! I call this my Magic Calorie Melt session because once you experience it you will witness the power of using your mind and body to make wiser choices and stay committed to your fitness goals and lifestyle.

The beauty of this practice is we just ease our way into complete relaxation, there is no pressure, no rush, and zero stress. That is where the magic happens! I will teach you how to relax completely, become still enough to listen to your body, and learn how to give it exactly the right amount of love and nourishment it needs. Before we begin, please find a peaceful spot where you are unlikely to be interrupted. Please switch all phones and doorbells to silent (if possible) or make sure you have headphones on. I need your full attention for you to gain the maximum benefits from this session.

I know you will really enjoy this session and soon start to look forward to the amazing ways your body will change. The weight will start to melt off and you will feel much lighter (in both mind, body, and spirit), you will look back in wonder at how effortless this process can be once you have the right tools, and you are equipped to make wiser, more mindful choices. (Pause). So now let us begin, get into a comfortable position, I like sitting back at a 45-degree angle against some comfy pillows or (in a comfortable chair). We want you comfortable but not likely to fall asleep so avoid laying down flat. (Pause).

I am about to take you on a truly mind-altering journey, stepping into your own power. All you need to do is chill! Know that you will learn many truths about your own mind and body on this journey. Your perceptions regarding food and exercise, your willpower and discipline levels all these things will shift massively, and you will witness mega results soon. (Pause). We are going to work on removing all the blocks from your path to fitness. Anything that slows you down has got to go. You will learn how to keep your equilibrium (balance) no matter what emotional stress or trigger occurs (and let us be honest, these are part of all our daily lives). (Pause). You will learn to recognize when you may be reaching for food as a comfort factor and reach for exercise instead. You will soon start to crave the buzz a great daily workout gives you (not to mention amazing beauty sleep). You will now know the secret to that sun-kissed glow so many celebrities and beauty icons wear with grace. (Pause).

Now let us start by gently taking three breaths. (Inhale gently and deeply, fill your stomach and lungs with air, hold for 2–3 seconds and release, exhale). (Wait for a few seconds to allow the reader to settle into the exercise).

Relax now and picture a giant jug with all your thoughts, worries, and fears. I will give you a few seconds, take everything that is currently in your mind, and put it into this jug.

(Pause allows 10–20 seconds). When you have emptied your mind, we will now begin our journey, all you need to do is listen to my voice, I will keep you safe and take you to a place of deep relaxation; that is where we get to work on our goals and melt off any unwanted weight (kilograms/ pounds).

Now I want you to imagine yourself feeling lighter and lighter. The more you relax, the lighter you feel. I want you to picture a beautiful winding stairway, can you see it? What color is it? Can you describe it a bit? (Pause). You are going to walk down those stairs on my count. (Slowly count down from 10 to 1).

You find yourself in front of a door built into a wall. (Pause) (You can start to play ocean-side music, waves gently caressing the sand) You can hear the ocean. You open the door and walk through it and find yourself face to face with the absolute beauty that is the ocean!

You take a minute to drink in the infinite beauty of the blue-green waves. You can smell the freshness and taste the salt in the air. Do you remember that big jug? We are going to empty it now into this ocean!

(Pause. Wait a few seconds until you follow this instruction mentally). Now that your mind is empty, I want you to fill it with the infinite wisdom from this ocean, with every inhalation, breathe in wisdom, and with every exhalation deepen your relaxation. (Pause). Now you should be in a state of complete chill; going deeper and deeper.

(Pause for a few seconds). You suddenly feel a familiar deep calm sensation, you remember what it is like to come home to yourself. You can feel yourself smiling, your heart is happy, this is the place you need to return to, to relax and peacefully, calmly focus on your weight loss journey.

You feel drawn closer to the ocean. You walk up to the water's edge and can feel the cool waves curling around your feet, giving you a deliciously cool tingle that relaxes you completely. You realize that this feeling returns you to your best self. You are now able to look at your weight loss goals and see where you need to make smarter choices. (Pause)

Suddenly you see that it just takes a few small changes in your food choices, a commitment to daily exercise, and the belief that you will achieve your fitness goals. That's all it will take to achieve your ideal weight and dream body. (Pause).

You now know that just like the ocean you may go through many phases, but you can always return to a state of tranquil beauty. The secret is knowing not to be too harsh with yourself. Do not beat yourself up. (Pause) Be kind to yourself, believe in yourself, stay committed (this means that even if you make a mistake one day, you forgive yourself and begin afresh the next) do not stop until all that weight has melted off. (Pause). You now start to feel really energized, the ocean breeze is invigorating, and you feel your energy levels returning to an optimal place. You suddenly feel the urge to go for a run/walk/jog.

And take off. You may run or walk briskly for a minute or 5, you may even make it through 20 mins. (Pause). You start to feel sweat gliding off you. You start to feel an ache in your legs. You feel like every part of your body is suddenly alive and in action.

You realize it feels so good. It aches in a good way, almost like a badge of honor, proof of your efforts. You earned this. You start to feel lighter and brighter and you feel so good, you realize you want to feel this way every day. So, you make a promise to yourself to work out like this at least 5–6 times a week. (Pause). It does not matter what form of cardio exercise you get; it does not matter whether it is indoors or outdoors, you can recreate this same image and relaxing feel anywhere!

You can see yourself waking up each day with a renewed sense of purpose and anticipation. You start to look forward to your day because each day you are growing slimmer and fitter. People are noticing and complimenting you. (Pause). You see yourself dropping dress sizes, looking fantastic in workout gear.

Your skin is glowing. You are eating healthier, choosing great foods that fill you up without making you feel lethargic. (Pause). You feel calmer now, more confident, excited even. You are aware of your breath and how important it is to breathe right. You realize that no matter what challenges and ups and downs you experience in your life every day, going forward you always have the choice to return to this place of calm and peace. (Pause).

You promise yourself that here on you will visit this place each day to strengthen your practice and reaffirm your goals. You now know that you no longer need to feel overwhelmed each time you can choose to return to your special place. You can choose to rejuvenate and replenish your energy and emotional levels right here. (Pause).

Knowing that it is perfectly safe and healthy, knowing that each time you choose to do this you grow lighter, more energized, healthier. (Pause) The fat is beginning to melt off now, you can feel it. All that excess weight literally just melting off. You are now drawn to walk a bit deeper into the ocean. The waves look so deliciously inviting that you choose to lie down and begin to float on your back. (Pause).

You begin to feel weightless for the first time and realize you love this feeling. As you float here, you feel so grateful to your body for carrying you so far! (Pause). Now you begin to scan it from head to toe, starting with your head, giving thanks for your ability to learn and grow wiser and make better choices regarding the food and drink you consume. (Pause).

You give thanks for your eyes. They have given you such different perspectives and allowed you to see that you do indeed have healthier options. (Pause). You give thanks to your nose and mouth; they help you to breathe correctly. (Pause). You give thanks for your heart, which fuels your entire body; you promise to exercise each day so you take the best care you possibly can of it. (Pause). You give thanks for your stomach and promise to be mindful of the food you put into it. (Pause). You give thanks for your hands and legs; they help you so much every day carrying your place, helping you get your work done. You promise to exercise them each day too. (Pause).

As you continue to float you realize this is easily the lightest you have ever felt. You are amazed and so grateful for this feeling and your newfound awareness. You have learned the benefits of exercise and had a glimpse of the new lighter you. You are just waiting to emerge. (Pause). You cannot wait to experience that feeling of freedom when you run or walk or jog. You will be one with nature, the lightness, the weightlessness, the satisfying ache that comes from working your body to its limits and enabling that fat to slide right off. You will revel in that floating sensation afterward. (Pause).

Now I am going to count down from ten and ask you to come back slowly to my voice and your surroundings. You may choose to rest for a while longer allowing your mind and body to absorb all your new learning and energy and ensure you continue to melt fat at all times (even whilst you are sleeping). (Pause). You may also choose to journal and write down how you feel after this hypnosis session. Ten. Nine. You feel so good. Eight. Seven, floating. Six. Five. Deeper still. Four. Three. That stubborn weight is just melting off. Two. One. You will melt fat all the time, even in your sleep.

Chapter 7 - Weight Loss Motivation Tips

• Surround yourself with people who have the same goals as you.

• Face your fears and take one step at a time.

• Take care of yourself by giving your body what it needs to stay healthy.

• Think about what will happen if you don't achieve your goal weight.

• Make a list of everything that triggers you to eat or drink nonstop. Identify the reasons why these things make you want to eat, drink, or do drugs more than usual and seek professional help for these triggers if necessary.

• Relapse (unknowingly) into old habits. Recognize the situation and think about how you will prevent it from ever happening again—this is a crucial step in successfully staying off the weight-loss wagon.

• Break bad habits with new ones that are healthier for your body.

• Take the time to eat and drink less while you're on the wagon.

• Diet coke is one of the worst things you could drink to lose weight, so make it a rule that you never drink diet coke again! You can replace diet soda with fruit-flavored waters or some sweet tea, but don't overdo the calories.

- Eat a low-calorie snack before dinner. That way you'll eat less and you'll be more satisfied with your meal.

- Drink lots of water and avoid carbonated drinks—they are full of sodium which causes you to retain water.

- Try not to shop when you're hungry. When you do go food shopping, take a snack such as an apple or carrot sticks along so that you won't "attack" the candy bars or chips when there's a free sample out on the counter!

- Remember why you started this journey in the first place and remind yourself every day what it feels like to be overweight.

- Visualize yourself at your goal weight.

- Work out, but don't overdo it and take frequent days off.

- Think about how awesome you'll feel when you reach your goal weight!

Chapter 8 - What Is Hypnotic Trance?

Hypnosis is a way of focusing your attention. By using guided relaxation techniques, you can learn to focus on the present moment and reduce distracting thoughts. Hypnotherapy is different as it uses the power of suggestion to help you change habits or beliefs which may be holding back your life.

Why Should I Use Hypnotic Trance?

It can help with: Stress management, pain relief, smoking cessation, weight management, phobias, and fears. Some people also use hypnotic trance for spiritual development such as past life regression and towards self-fulfillment goals such as healing connections or gaining insights from past experiences in other lives by using past life regression Practitioners.

What Are the Benefits of Hypnotic Trance?

Hypnosis can help you to focus and relax in a deep trance state. You can use this time of peace and quiet to manage stress and tension. Using state-specific suggestions, you may be able to overcome fears and phobias or stop smoking. Hypnotic trance can also be used as a learning tool for the techniques of hypnosis.

Hypnotherapy uses the power of suggestion during hypnosis training sessions in order to change old beliefs that may be holding you back from living your life to its fullest potential. You can purchase the audio course at iTunes or Google play store. Our Hypnotherapy Masters Hypnosis

Course includes a full education on hypnosis including methods of induction, deepening techniques, suggestions, and how to track your progress. Hypnotic trance can help you to:

- **Manage stress levels and achieve the relaxation you need!** When you are in a deep hypnotic trance, you can focus all your attention on the present moment. Using the power of suggestion, you can reduce distracting thoughts, make positive changes to your beliefs and behaviors that empower you and help you relax.

- **Make changes and achieve new life goals!** Hypnotherapy can be used to make changes that will help you to be the best person you can possibly be. You can change old habits, beliefs, and behaviors that may be holding you back. Hypnosis allows you to bypass your conscious mind and make positive changes in order to move forward with your life. You can also use hypnotherapy as a tool for learning how to produce a hypnotic trance state on your own. Through regular practice, you can gain mastery over the art of self-hypnosis.

State of Hypnotic Trance vs. the State of Meditation

People often believe that hypnosis is a type of meditation. This is not true, as meditation has different goals, which are usually in the pursuit of personal development, spiritual peace, relaxation, and well-being. Hypnosis has a very different objective; to help someone accept a suggestion to change their behavior in order to achieve some goal.

Meditation can be used by anyone for relaxation, personal development, and stress management including self-hypnosis but it is usually not used as a tool for making changes in life by using self-hypnosis and hypnotic trance. Most people who use meditation do not use it as a way to change beliefs or behavior because they have found that it does not work for them.

If you are interested in self-hypnosis and trance meditation, it is recommended that you learn how to use trance meditation for personal development rather than hypnosis, which is a method of self-hypnosis. Using trance meditation will help you to be able to achieve goals that involve personal development.

How to Use Self-Hypnosis to Make Changes in the Present Moment?

The feeling of relaxation comes from very deep within you; however, it can feel like a very distant experience if your mind is distracted by thoughts or concerns. When these unwanted thoughts come into your mind, remember to relax and let them go because they are not needed when using self-hypnosis and trance meditation techniques.

Chapter 9 - Understanding Food Addictions

Addictions have a way of tricking the mind and body into thinking that they are normal, but in reality, most are actually maladaptive struggles. A good example of this is food addiction. The term "food addiction" has been thrown around so often that people may not even know what it means or how to overcome it. Let's take a moment to break down the meaning of "food addiction" and explore some treatment options for overcoming their struggles with this type of addictive behavior.

What Exactly Is Food Addiction?

Food addiction—also referred to as compulsive eating, refeeding syndrome, and eating disorder not otherwise specified (EDNOS)—is a type of substance or behavior addiction that involves an obsession with food. The food may not be in excess, but there is an unhealthy pattern of binging and purging that occurs on a regular basis. Some common symptoms include:

• **Eating a lot more than normal:** You're often hungry after you eat.

• **Eating quickly:** You eat large amounts of food in a short period of time.

• **Bingeing when you eat:** You end up eating huge amounts of food to the point where you feel extremely full or sick afterward.

- **Not being able to stop eating:** You can't stop eating, even if you are not hungry.

- **Eating to deal with boredom:** You binge when you are bored, lonely, or depressed.

- **Eating to control your emotions:** You binge when you feel stressed, angry, or anxious.

Although there is no official medical diagnosis for food addiction that includes every symptom that might present with the condition, some other criteria such as weight gain and a pattern of irregular eating habits could be used to diagnose this problem. In most cases of food addiction, though, the behavior does not cause serious harm toward other people or yourself; however, it can still ruin a person's quality of life if they don't find a way to overcome it.

What Causes Food Addiction?

Food addiction can be caused by a person's environment, genetic profile, and/or mental health. The following are examples of how these three categories of influence may lead to food addiction:

- **Environmental factors:** Food addiction can be caused by an environment that promotes unhealthy eating habits. For example, it is not uncommon for a person living in poverty to live in an area where inexpensive, processed foods are readily available. It is also possible that the person has no time or energy to cook healthier meals on a daily basis. This could lead to the consumption of highly processed and sugary foods that eventually ruin their health.

276

- **Genetic profile:** A person's genetic profile may also play a role in food addiction, as certain types of substances and behaviors may run in their family. For example, if one parent struggles with alcoholism, there is a possibility that the child may experience some level of alcohol addiction at some point in life. It may seem like it is an issue of the child's own making, but there is clearly a genetic component to this kind of addiction.

- **Mental health issues:** A person's mental health could play a role as well. Many people with depression or anxiety disorders have an unhealthy relationship with food that makes it more difficult for them to eat well-balanced meals on a regular basis. They may rely on food for comfort when they feel stressed or anxious, which eventually leads to a reliance on the mood-altering properties of food.

Early Signs of Food Addiction

Although there is no specific list of early signs of food addiction, watching out for the following behaviors can help you determine if you have an unhealthy relationship with food:

- **Mood swings and emotional eating:** Mood swings are normal during moments when you are stressed or anxious. However, there is a difference between experiencing a temporary drop in mood and allowing it to affect your eating habits. In an unhealthy relationship with food, a person will binge eat when they experience stress or anxiety. This can become so ingrained in their behavior that it may be difficult to break the cycle on their own.

- **Overeating or undereating:** Overeating or undereating are both examples of unhealthy eating habits that could lead to food addiction. For example, if you overeat, you may feel guilty for your actions and purge afterward. If you undereat, you may feel ashamed for not being able to meet your nutritional needs and binge eat as a result.

- **Body image issues:** A person who struggles with the way they look is prone to experience problems surrounding food in some way or another. This is especially true when they overeat or undereat because of their lack of self-love.

- **Spending money on foods:** If you regularly spend more money than you can afford on foods, this may be a sign that you have developed an unhealthy relationship with food.

Although there are no clear clinical symptoms of food addiction that can be used to diagnose the condition, it is possible to detect an irregular eating pattern that makes it difficult for a person to lead a healthy lifestyle. The good news is that food addiction is 100% treatable with effective medical intervention and psychotherapeutic support. The most important thing is to reach out for help if you feel like your eating behaviors are becoming a problem in your life.

Treatment Options

There are many treatment options available to help you overcome an unhealthy relationship with food. The following are some of the most effective treatment strategies:

- **Cognitive-behavioral therapy (CBT):** CBT can be used for a variety of eating disorders and other mental health conditions, including food addiction. It encourages individuals to make more conscious choices about their dietary habits by making sure that they are eating balanced meals that promote good health. It also teaches them better coping skills so they can manage their stress and anxiety without turning to food as a solution.

• **Group therapy:** Group therapy can be helpful for people who are dealing with an addictive relationship with food. This type of group therapy promotes healthy eating habits through role-playing, developing healthier nutritional goals, and helping them identify the negative thought patterns that may be driving their problematic eating habits.

• **Individual therapy:** Individual therapy can be extremely helpful for those in recovery from food addiction. It allows them to work on their issues in a private and confidential setting, so they do not have to worry about how other people are responding to their behaviors.

• **Medication:** If you are experiencing an unhealthy relationship with food and struggle to break free on your own, it may be time to explore a medication option. In some cases, medications can help reduce the cravings involved with an addictive relationship with food.

• **Nutritional counseling:** Nutritional counseling is another effective way to aid in the recovery process for someone who is struggling with food addiction. It can help you develop a healthier relationship with food by addressing your cravings and unhelpful thoughts.

• **Psychotropic medication:** Certain medications used to treat behavioral addictions, such as mood stabilizers, may be helpful if you are dealing with an eating disorder and struggle with inappropriate eating behaviors as well.

- **Transference therapy:** Transference therapy is an approach that aims to help clients identify any emotional or mental traumas that may have been influenced by the addictive relationship they developed with food in the past.

- **Yoga:** Yoga is a popular form of relaxation therapy that tends to help people overcome food addiction. It can aid in the transformation process by allowing you to clear your mind of negative thoughts and feelings and develop healthier eating habits.

Although there are no easy or fast solutions for overcoming an addiction to unhealthy food, it is important that you seek out the help you need as soon as possible. There are countless resources available for those who have made this difficult decision so they can begin the journey to recovery and a better quality of life.

Chapter 10 - When the Mind Affects Our Weight and Choice of Food

When you are trying to lose weight, you need to know what you're up against. Your mind should be your top ally, but many people fight viciously against their minds in the battle of the bulge, and they make it even harder to lose weight. The human mind is a remarkable organ with capacities that we haven't even begun to unlock, but neuroscience and psychology can help us understand the basic, instinctual powers of the brain. I've already deliberated basic ideas of how the unconscious brain works and how it can lead you to reach your goals, but beyond the scientific elements, you need to understand how your specific mind functions because while brains function in similar ways, experiences, and biology shift how you think. Know the things that give you the most trouble. Everyone has problem areas.

Maybe you love ice cream, and if there is ice cream in the house, you can't stay away from it. In this case, pay special attention to that craving. Don't cut ice cream out of your diet entirely, but it would help to limit how much temptation you keep around. Similarly, if you have trouble finding time for exercise, make sure you take extra efforts to carve out space for some physical activity. Acknowledge the parts of losing weight that is hardest for you, and act accordingly.

Recognize what you've done wrong in the past when you've tried to lose weight. You've probably tried to lose weight before. Most people have, so reflect upon those experiences, and try to figure out what you did wrong then.

Maybe you weren't in the right headspace then. Maybe you didn't have the tools you needed for success. Whatever the problem was, find ways to avoid that problem, and be realistic with yourself. Don't fool yourself into thinking you can do better this time by using sheer willpower. People can change, but change isn't just going to happen, so work within your current limits and then expand your boundaries as you go.

• **Know what you're good at.** Don't neglect to pay attention to the things you do well in your weight loss journey. These things are what you should hold onto from past diets. Your skills can be used to further your success. Don't let them set in the corner of your mind, dusty and untouched. Embrace those skills and use them as fully as you possibly can because that will give you the greatest results, and it will make you feel happier because ginormous amounts of satisfaction come with doing things that you're good at.

• **Understand your limits.** Know what you cannot do. If you can't cut out your morning bowl of sugary cereal without freaking out and binging in the evening, then don't. Maybe someday you'll be able to gradually get rid of that cereal, maybe you won't. We all have our limits and things that we simply aren't willing to change at this moment. Don't force the change. Find ways to work within your limits. You may have to use a little imagination, but with careful attention, your limits don't have to limit your progress.

• **Check your doubts.** If you doubt that you can do this or that you should do this, learn to speak up against those doubts. Doubt can be very nasty and tell you that you're not worth the change or that you're a lost cause. Don't listen to those doubts. Remind yourself of why that doubt is wrong. Think extremely hard about it, and you can probably find a few

282

reasons why the voice in your head is wrong. Acknowledge also that sometimes your doubts are right. For example, when you doubt that an extreme-sounding diet will benefit you, you're probably right. If you're making dietary decisions out of desperation rather than thoughtfulness, you may want to listen to that doubt.

- **Doubt doesn't have to be your enemy.** It has incredibly good input sometimes, but you don't have to blindly believe your doubts either.

- **Focus on forever, not just now.** When things get tough, think of all the things you hope for in the future. Visualize who you want to be and use that visualization as motivation to carry on through the hardest parts of your journey. You and your body will be forever tied together. You can't move your brain to a new body, so make the best of the relationship between your body and mind. Let your dreams connect the two and let yourself be hopeful for what is to come. There's no need to be afraid of your hopes. There's nothing wrong with expecting the best, even if you don't quite reach those hopes.

- **Don't let the past drag you back.** Whatever challenges you've faced in the past or insecurities, you don't have to let those things dictate who you are now. Your past pains and joys shape you as a person. You can't outrun your trauma, but you don't have to let it continue to hurt you. The future is yours for the taking, and you can shape it into whatever you want. There is happiness there, but you have to build it for yourself, even with the cruel aspects of the world.

- **Don't forget to find things that give you joy.** The things that make you happy are more important than ever. These are the things that are going to get you through, and you can find joy by doing things you

283

love, but you can also take this moment to try new things. New experiences can both be motivating and exciting. Thus, they can give your mind something else to focus on if you get too fixated on losing weight. You need recreation in your life. If you just work all the time, you get stressed and become unable to succeed, so relaxation doesn't just make you feel better, it changes how well you will be able to make the needed changes.

• **Keep yourself incentivized.** Rewards for your progress and your efforts. Use rewards that aren't related to food. Buy yourself something nice or take a day off work to do something you enjoy. Give yourself all the motivation that you need to create change and feel excited about the future and all it holds.

Weight loss is grueling, but knowing who you're up against is one of the best tools you can have. Weight loss is an internal battle, which can be one of the hardest types of battles that you'll ever fight, but if you learn about yourself and know your strengths and shortcomings, you can master weight loss and get the most out of hypnosis. A little self-discovery can go a long way, and I urge you to continue to learn about yourself throughout this journey. Get to know the person you are as well as the person you are becoming for the best results.

Chapter 11 - Psychology of Emotional Eating

We will look more in-depth at emotional eating to give you more information about what it is, why it occurs, and what could cause it. We will begin by once again defining emotional eating. Emotional eating occurs when a person suffering from emotional deficiencies of some sort including lack of affection, lack of connection, or other factors like stress, depression, anxiety, or even general negative feelings like sadness or anger, eats or gives into food cravings that occur as a result of these emotional deficiencies to achieve feelings of comfort from the food they are eating.

How Food Cravings Can Indicate Emotional Deficiencies

You may be asking how food cravings can result from emotional deficiencies and how these two seemingly unrelated things can be considered related. The reason for this is that your body over time learns that eating certain foods like those containing processed sugars or salts like fast food and quick pastries makes it feel rewarding, positive, and happy for some time after it is ingested.

When you are sad or worried, your body feels down and looks for ways to remedy this. Your brain then connects these two facts and decides that eating these foods will make it feel better. As a result of this process that happens in the background without you being aware of it, you then consciously feel a craving for those foods like sugary snacks or salty fast-food meals, and you may not even be aware of why. If you later decide to give in to this craving and eat something like a microwave pizza snack, your body will feel rewarded and happy for a brief time, which reinforces to your brain that craving food to make itself feel better emotionally has worked. If you end up feeling down and guilty that you ate something that was unhealthy, your brain will again try to remedy these negative emotions by craving food, and a cycle of emotional eating can then begin without you being any the wiser.

Below is a visual display of the period of emotional eating.

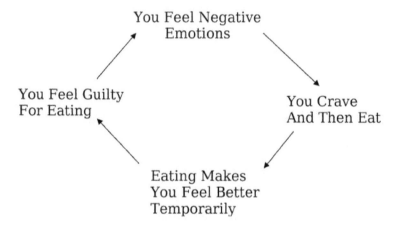

The Cycle of Emotional Eating

Because scientists and psychiatrists understand this process that occurs in the brain, they know that food cravings can indicate emotional deficiencies.

While other types of desires can occur, such as those that pregnant ladies experience or those that show nutrient deficiencies, there are ways to tell that a need is caused by emotional lacking of some sort. It begins by determining the foods that a person craves and when they want them. If every time someone has a stressful situation, they feel like eating a pizza, or if a person who is depressed tends to eat much chocolate, this could indicate emotional eating. If you crave fruits like a watermelon on a hot day, you are likely just dehydrated, and your body is trying to get water from a water-filled fruit that it knows will make it more hydrated. Examining things and situations like his leads scientists and psychiatrists to explore this concept in more depth and determine what types of emotional deficiencies can manifest themselves through food cravings in this way. We will look closer at these specific emotional deficiencies.

Examples of Emotional Deficiencies

There are several types of emotional deficiencies that can be indicated by food cravings. We will explore these in detail below in hopes that you will recognize some of the reasons why you may experience struggles with eating.

Childhood Causes

The first example of an emotional deficiency that we will examine is more of an umbrella for various psychological defects. This umbrella term is Childhood Causes. If you think back on your childhood, think about how your relationship with food was cultivated. Maybe you were taught that when you behaved, you received food as a reward. Maybe when you were feeling down, you were given food to cheer you up. Perhaps you turned to food when you were experiencing negative things in your childhood. Any of these could cause someone to suffer from emotional eating in their adulthood, as it had become something learned. This type is quite challenging to break as it has likely been a habit for many, many years, but it is possible. When we are children, we learn habits and make associations without knowing it that we often carry into our later lives.

Covering up Emotions

Another emotional deficiency that can manifest itself in emotional eating and food cravings is the effort to cover up our emotions. Sometimes we would somewhat distract ourselves and cover up our feelings than feel them or face them head-on. In this case, our brain may make us feel hungry to distract us from the act of eating food. When we have a quiet minute where these feelings or thoughts would pop into our minds, we can cover them up by deciding to prepare food and eat, and convince ourselves that we are "too busy" to acknowledge our feelings because we have to deal with our hunger.

The fact that it is the hunger that arises in this scenario makes it very difficult to ignore and very easy to deem as a necessary distraction since, after all, we do need to eat to survive. This can be a problem, though, if we do not need nourishment, and we are telling ourselves that this is the reason why we cannot deal with our demons or our emotions.

Feeling Empty or Bored

When we feel bored, we often decide to eat or decide that we are hungry. This occupies our mind and our time and makes us feel less fatigued and even feel positive and happy. We also may eat when we are feeling empty.

288

When we feel empty, the food will quite literally be ingested to fill a void, but as we know, the feed will not fill a void that is emotional in sort, and this will lead to an unhealthy cycle of trying to fill orselves emotionally with something that will never actually work. This will lead us to become disappointed every time and continue trying to fill this void with material things like food or purchases. This can also be a general feeling of dissatisfaction with life and opinions of lacking something in your life.

Looking deeper into this the next time you feel those cravings will be severe but will help you greatly in the long term as you will then be able to identify the source of your feelings of emptiness and begin to fill these voids in ways that will be much more effective.

Affection Deficiency

Another emotional deficiency that could manifest itself as food cravings is an affection deficiency. This type of weakness can be feelings of loneliness, emotions of a lack of love, or feelings of being undesired. If a person has been without an intimate relationship or has recently gone through a breakup, or if a person has not experienced physical intimacy in quite some time, they may be experiencing an affection deficiency. This type of emotional weakness will often manifest itself in food cravings, as we will try to gain feelings of comfort and positivity from the excellent tasting, drug-like foods they crave.

Low Self-Esteem

Another emotional deficiency that may be indicated by food cravings is a low level of self-esteem. Low self-esteem can cause people to feel down, unlovable, inadequate, and overall negative and sad. This can make a person feel like eating foods they enjoy will make them feel better, even if only for a few moments. Low self-esteem is an emotional deficiency that is difficult to deal with as it affects every area of a person's life, such as their love life, their social life, their career life, and so on. Sometimes people have reported feeling like food was something that was always there for them, and that never left them. While this is true, they will often be left feeling even emptier and lower about themselves after giving into cravings.

Mood

A general low mood can cause emotional eating. While the problem of emotional eating is something that is occurring multiple times per week and we all have general depressed feelings or bad days, if this makes you crave food and especially food of an unhealthy sort, this could become emotional eating. If every time we feel down or are having a bad day, we want to eat food to make ourselves feel better; this is emotional eating. Some people will have a bad day and want a drink at the end of the day, and if this happens every once in a while, it is not necessarily a problem with emotional eating.

The more often it happens, the more often it is emotional eating. Further, we do not have to give in to the cravings for it to be considered emotional eating. Experiencing the needs often and in tandem with negative feelings in the first place is what constitutes emotional eating.

Depression

Suffering from depression also can lead to emotional eating. Depression is a constant low mood for a period of months on end, and this depressed mood can cause a person to turn to food for comfort and a lift in spirit. This can then become emotional eating in addition to and because of depression.

Anxiety

Having anxiety can lead to emotional eating as well. There are several types of concern, and whether it is general anxiety (constant levels of stress), situational anxiety (triggered by a situation or scenario), it can lead to emotional eating. You have likely heard of the term comfort food to describe certain foods and dishes. The reason for this is that they are usually foods rich in carbohydrates, fats, and cumbersome in nature. These foods bring people a sense of comfort. These foods are often turned to when people suffering from anxiety are emotionally eating because these foods help to ease their stress temporarily and make them feel calmer and more at ease.

This only lasts for a short time; however, before their anxiety usually gears up again.

Stress

Stress eating is probably the most common form of emotional eating. While this does not become an issue for everyone experiencing stress, and many people will do so every once in a while, it is a problem for those who consistently turn to food to ease their burden. Some people are always under pressure, and they will continuously be looking for ways to alleviate their anxiety. Food is one of these ways that people use to make themselves feel better and to take their minds off of their importance. As with all the other examples we have seen above, this is not a lasting resolution, and it becomes a cycle. Similar to the cycle diagram we saw above, the same can be used for stress except instead of negative emotion and eating making you feel more down, stress eating can make you feel more pressure as you feel like you have done something you shouldn't have which causes you to stress, and the cycle ensues.

Chapter 12 - Why Do People Fail to Lose Weight?

You can say goodbye to obsessing over your daily calorie intake and the carbohydrates you have eaten today. You can say goodbye to extremely restrictive bans on foods as well as on other forced behaviors in pursuance of focusing on getting back into shape in a healthy, natural way by following your body's biology.

You have probably blamed yourself, or your lack of self-discipline, in the past. You probably have blamed calories and your dieting formulas, which most certainly did not bring anything good your way. The truth is that there is no one and nothing to blame here. Every step you have taken in the past can teach you something which will help you to succeed in the future.

Another truth is that losing weight can be an extremely difficult thing to do and there are different reasons behind this. If you are focused on the weight loss industry, you have probably been told many times before how easy it is to shed those additional pounds.

The industry generally suggests you take this pill, drink that beverage, or buy this equipment and simply enjoy your additional pounds melting on their own. The truth is that the industry generates billions of dollars every year thanks to individuals who spend their money on different weight loss tools and products which can only be effective in the short run. Accordingly, many people struggling with weight are still overweight despite hundreds of dollars spent in the industry.

Now, you probably wonder why it is so hard and challenging to lose those additional pounds. It should be noted that there is no magical pill, magical tool, or magical equipment that can make the process runs smoothly.

Dieting plans that suggest you completely change your dieting pattern, quit eating your favorite foods and similar restrictions do not work. There is also scientific evidence as clear as it can get that suggests that cutting your daily calorie intake will not by any means lead to health gains or long-term weight loss.

It would be logical that most dieters have realized they have wrong dieting patterns, but still, individuals set those same weight goals every year.

The truth is that dieting failures are the norm. There is also a massive stigma surrounding heavier people and, on many occasions, we can witness the massive blame game which is directed towards dieters who are not able to shed those additional pounds.

On the other hand, looking from a scientific point of view, it is clear that dieting most certainly sets up a truly unfair fight.

Many people are confused to learn of diet plans that suggest extreme changes, but this only comes as a result of statements that do not square with their previous observations.

Some thin people consume junk food and still stay thin without their food choices affecting their weight. These people most usually think that they stay in shape due to their dieting habits, but the truth is that genetics plays a massive role in helping them stay fit. These people are praised for their dieting choices, as others can only see what they consume, but they cannot examine what is inside their genes.

The Importance of Genetics

Due to the role of genetics, many individuals struggling with excess pounds will not be as thin as other people even if they embrace the same dieting choices as them and consume them in the exact same quantities.

The bodies of those heavier people can run on fewer calories than thin people require, which may sound like a promising thing.

On the other hand, this means that they have more calories left, stored as fat in the body after eating the same food in the same quantities as thinner people.

This means that they need to consume fewer foods than thin people in order to shed pounds. Once they have followed some dieting plan for some time, their overall metabolic state changes so they need to consume even fewer calories in pursuance of losing further weight. It isn't only genetics that makes thin people stay thin, but it is also their mindset revolving around dieting and fitness.

For thin people, as they are non-dieters, it is very easy to ignore those sugary treats and desserts which for heavier people seem like a massive challenge and obstacle on their weight loss journey.

For heavier people, these treats and sugary candies seem as if they are almost jumping around cheerfully making them approach and eat them.

This being said, dieting of any kind causes specific neurological changes which make people more likely to be focused on foods and notice foods everywhere. Once they notice foods, those neurological changes happening in the brain are what make it almost impossible to not think about food.

Thin people often forget those sweets on the desk, but dieters tend to keep obsessing over them. As a matter of fact, dieters seem to crave these foods even more due to those neurological changes.

Moreover, these neurological changes make food taste better due to the fact they cause a greater rush of dopamine or the reward hormone.

This is the same hormone released when drug addicts or substance abusers use their drugs. Individuals who are non-dieters do not suffer from these kinds of rushes, so they can peacefully leave a piece of cake untouched.

Dieters also tend to struggle with another issue revolving around neurological changes that affect their hormonal balance.

They face another uphill battle when their leptin hormone or satiety hormone levels go down. Due to this hormonal change, dieters require even more foods to consume in pursuance of feeling full.

This means that they felt hungry following their dieting plans and over some time they feel even hungrier once again due to hormonal changes.

Chapter 13 - Step by Step Guide to Hypnotherapy for Weight Loss

1. **Believe.** A significant part of the intensity of spellbinding lies in your conviction that you have a method for assuming responsibility for your desires. If you don't figure entrancing will enable you to change your emotions, it will probably have little impact.

2. **Become agreeable.** Go to a spot where you may not be stressed. This can resemble your bed, a couch, or a pleasant, comfortable chair anyplace. Ensure you bolster your head and neck. Wear loose garments and ensure the temperature is set at an agreeable level. It might be simpler to unwind if you play some delicate music while mesmerizing yourself, particularly something instrumental.

3. **Focus on an item.** Discover something to take a gander at and focus on in the room, ideally something somewhat above you. Utilize your concentration for clearing your leader of all contemplations on this item. Make this article the main thing that you know about.

4. **Breathing is crucial.** When you close your eyes, inhale profoundly. Reveal to yourself the greatness of your eyelids and let them fall delicately. Inhale profoundly with an ordinary mood as your eyes close. Concentrate on your breathing, enabling it to assume control over your whole personality, much like the item you've been taking a gander at previously. Feel progressively loose with each fresh breath. Envision that your muscles disperse all the pressure and stress. Permit this inclination from your face, your chest, your arms, lastly, your legs to descend your

body. When you're entirely loose, your psyche should be clear, and you will be a self-mesmerizing piece.

5. **Display a pendulum.** Customarily, the development of a pendulum moving to and from has been utilized to energize the center is spellbinding. Picture this pendulum in your psyche, moving to and from. Concentrate on it as you unwind to help clear your brain.

6. **Start by focusing on 10 to 1 in your mind.** You advise yourself as you check down that you are steadily getting further into entrancing. State: 10, I'm alleviating. 9, I get increasingly loose. 8. I can feel my body spreading unwinding. 7, Nothing yet unwinding I can feel.... 1, I'm resting profoundly. Keep in mind that you will be in a condition of spellbinding when you accomplish 1 all through.

7. **Waking up from self-hypnosis.** Once, during spellbinding, you have accomplished what you need, you should wake up. From 1 to 10, check back. State in your mind: 1, I wake up. 2, I'll feel like I woke up from a significant rest when I tally down. 3, I feel wakeful more.... 10, I'm wakeful, and I'm new.

8. **Develop a plan.** Reinventing your mind with spellbinding requires consistent redundancy. You ought to endeavor in a condition of spellbinding to go through around twenty minutes per day. While beneath, shift back and forth between portions of the underneath referenced methodologies. Attempt to assault your poor eating rehearses from any edge.

9. **Learn to refrain from emotional overeating.** One of the main things you should endeavor to do under mesmerizing is to influence yourself. You are not intrigued by the frightful nibble of food you

298

experience issues kicking. Pick something that you will, in general, revel in like frozen yogurt. State, "Dessert tastes poor and makes me feel debilitated." Repeat twenty minutes until you're prepared to wake up from the trance. Keep in mind; excellent eating regimen doesn't suggest you have to quit eating, simply eat less awful sustenance. Simply influence yourself to devour less food, you know, is undesirable.

10.   **Write your very own positive mantra.** Self-spellbinding ought to be utilized to reinforce your longing to eat better. Compose a mantra to rehash in a trance state. It harms me and my body when I overeat.

11.   **Imagine the best thing for you.** Picture what you might want to be more beneficial to support your longing to live better. From when you were slenderer, take a picture of yourself or do your most extreme to figure what you'd resemble in the wake of shedding pounds. Concentrate on this image under mesmerizing. Envision the trust you'd feel on the off chance that you'd be more advantageous. This will cause you to comprehend that when you wake up. Eat each supper with protein. Protein is especially valuable at topping you off and can improve your digestion since it advances muscle improvement. Fish, lean meat, eggs, yogurt, nuts, and beans are great wellsprings of protein. A steak each dinner might be counterproductive, yet in case you're eager, eating on nuts could go far to helping you accomplish your objectives.

12.   **Eat a few, modest meals daily.** If you don't eat for quite a while, your digestion will go down, and you will stop fat consumption. If you expend something modest once every three or four hours, your metabolism will go up, and when you plunk down for dinner, you will be less hungry.

13.   **Eat organically grown foods.** You will be loaded up with foods grown from the ground and furnish you with supplements without putting any pounds on. To start shedding pounds, nibble on bananas rather than treats to quicken weight reduction.

14.   **Cut down on unhealthy fats.** It tends to be helpful for you to have unsaturated fats, similar to those in olive oil. Nonetheless, you should endeavor to limit your saturated fat and trans-fat intake. Both of these are significant factors that add to coronary illness.

13.   **Learn more about healthy cooking.** In preparing meals, trans fats are common, mainly when eating meals, sweets, and fast food.

14.   **Saturated fats may not be as bad as trans fats.** However, they might be undesirable. Primary saturated fat sources include spreads, cheddar cheese, grease, red meat, and milk. The journey to weight loss is not an easy one. A person needs a lot of help and motivation to succeed. With the help of hypnotherapy, one can easily stay the course and watch the pounds melt away. Following the guide above and with a credible hypnotherapist or mastering self-hypnosis will help you achieve your goals.

Chapter 14 - Mindful Eating Habits
Understanding Mindful Eating

There are various scopes of cautious eating techniques, some of them established in Zen and different kinds of Buddhism, others connected to yoga. Here, we are taking a simple technique, and that is the primary concern we're going to discuss in this. My careful eating procedure is figuring out how to be cautious. Rather than eating carelessly, putting nourishment unknowingly in your mouth, not so much tasting the sustenance you eat, you see your thoughts and feelings.

- **Learn to be cautious:** why you want to eat, and what emotions or requirements can trigger eating.

- What you eat, and whether it's solid.

- Look, smell, taste, feel the nourishment that you eat.

- How do you feel when you taste it, how would you digest it, and go about your day?

- How complete you are previously, during, and in the wake of eating.

- During and in the wake of eating, your sentiments.

- Where the nourishment originated from, who could have developed it, the amount it could have suffered before it was killed, regardless of whether it was naturally developed, the amount it was handled, the amount it was broiled or overcooked, and so on.

This is an ability that you don't simply increase medium-term, a type of reflection. It takes practice, and there will be times when you neglect to eat mindfully, beginning, and halting. However, you can get generally excellent at this with exercise and consideration.

Mindful Eating Benefits

The upsides of eating mindfully are unimaginable and realizing these points of interest is fundamental as you think about the activity.

• When you're anxious, you figure out how to eat and stop when you're plunking down.

• You figure out how to taste nourishment and acknowledge great sustenance tastes.

• You start to see gradually that unfortunate nourishment isn't as scrumptious as you accepted, nor does it make you feel extremely pleasant.

• Because of the over three points, if you are overweight, you will regularly get more fit.

• You start arranging your nourishment and eating through the passionate issues you have. It requires somewhat more, yet it's basic.

• Social overeating can turn out to be less of an issue—you can eat mindfully while mingling, rehearsing, and not over-alimenting.

• You begin to appreciate the experience of eating more, and as an outcome, you will acknowledge life more when you are progressively present.

- It can transform into a custom of mindfulness that you anticipate.

- You learn for the day how nourishment impacts your disposition and vitality.

- You realize what fuels your training best with nourishment, and you work and play.

A Guide to Mindful Eating

Keeping up a contemporary, quick-paced way of life can leave a brief period to oblige your necessities. You are moving, always starting with one thing, and then onto the next, not focusing on what your psyche or body truly needs.

Rehearsing mindfulness can help you to comprehend those necessities. When eating mindfulness is connected, it can help you recognize your examples and practices while simultaneously standing out to appetite and completion related to body signs.

Originating from the act of pressure decrease dependent on mindfulness, rehearsing mindfulness while eating can help you focus on the present minute instead of proceeding with ongoing and unacceptable propensities. Careful eating is an approach to begin an internal looking course to help you become increasingly aware of your nourishment association and utilize that information to eat with joy.

The body conveys a great deal of information and information, so you can start settling on cognizant choices as opposed to falling into programmed—and regularly feeling-driven—practices when you apply attention to the eating knowledge. You are better prepared to change your conduct once you become aware of these propensities.

Individuals that need to be cautious about sustenance and nourishment are asked to:

•   Explore their inward knowledge about sustenance—different preferences.

•   Choose foods that please and support their bodies.

•   Accept explicit sustenance inclinations without judgment or self-analysis.

•   Practice familiarity with the indications of their bodies beginning to eat and quit eating.

General Principles of Mindful Eating

One methodology for careful eating depends on the core values given by Rebecca J. Frey, Ph.D., and Laura Jean Cataldo, RN: tune in to the internal craving and satiety signs of your body identify private triggers for careless eating, for example, social weights, amazing sentiments, and explicit nourishments. Here are a couple of tips for getting you started:

•   **Start with one meal.** It requires some investment to begin with any new propensity. It very well may be difficult to make cautious eating rehearses constantly. However, you can practice with one dinner or even a segment of a supper. Attempt to focus on appetite sign and sustenance choices before you start eating or sinking into the feelings of satiety toward the part of the arrangement—these are phenomenal approaches to begin a routine with regards to consideration.

- **Remove view distractions off your phone in another space.** Mood killers such as TV and PC and set away whatever else —for example, books, magazines, and papers—that can divert you from eating. Give the feast before your complete consideration.

- **Tune in your perspective when you start this activity, become aware of your attitude.** Perceive that there is no right or off base method for eating, yet simply unmistakable degrees of eating background awareness. Focus your consideration on eating sensations. When you understand that your brain has meandered, take it delicately back to the eating knowledge.

- **Draw in your senses with this activity.** There are numerous approaches to explore. Attempt to investigate one nourishment thing utilizing every one of your faculties. When you put sustenance in your mouth, see the scents, surfaces, hues, and flavors. Attempt to see how the sustenance changes as you cautiously bite each nibble.

- **Take as much time as necessary.** Eating cautiously includes backing off, enabling your stomach-related hormones to tell your mind that you are finished before eating excessively. It's a fabulous method to hinder your fork between chomps. Additionally, you will be better arranged to value your supper experience, especially in case you're with friends and family.

- Rehearsing mindfulness in a bustling globe can be trying now and again; however, by knowing and applying these essential core values and

305

techniques, you can discover approaches to settle your body all the more promptly. When you figure out how much your association with nourishment can adjust to improve things, you will be charmingly astounded—and this can importantly affect your general prosperity and well-being.

Formal dinners, be that as it may, will, in general, assume a lower priority about occupied ways of life for general people. Rather, supper times are an opportunity to endeavor to do each million stuff in turn. Consider having meals at your work area or accepting your Instagram fix over breakfast to control a task. The issue with this is you are bound to be genuinely determined in your decisions about healthy eating and eat excessively on the off chance that you don't focus on the nourishment you devour or the way you eat it.

That is the place mindfulness goes in. You can apply similar plans to a yoga practice straight on your lunch plate. "Cautious eating can enable you to tune in to the body's information of what, when, why, and the amount to eat," says Lynn Rossy, Ph.D., essayist of The Mindfulness-Based Eating Solution and the Center for Mindful Eating director. "Rather than relying upon another person (or an eating routine) to reveal to you how to eat, developing a minding association with your own body can achieve tremendous learning and change."

From the ranch to the fork—can help you conquer enthusiastic eating, make better nourishment choices, and even experience your suppers in a crisp and ideally better way. To make your next dinner mindful, pursue these measures.

The most effective method to Start Eating More Intentionally

- **Stage 1—Eat before you shop.** We have all been there. You go with a rumbling stomach to the shop. You meander the passageways, and out of the blue, those power bars and microwaveable suppers start to look truly enticing. "When you're excessively ravenous, shopping will, in general, shut us off from our progressively talented goals of eating in a way that searches useful for the body," says Dr. Rossy. So, even if you feel the slightest craving or urge to eat, get a nutritious bite or a light meal before heading out. That way, your food choices will be made intentionally when you shop, as opposed to propelled by craving or an unexpected sugar crash in the blood.

- **Stage 2—Make conscious food choices.** When you truly start considering where your nourishment originates from, you're bound to pick sustenance that is better for you. The earth and people busy with the expansion procedure portrays Meredith Klein, a canny kitchen educator and author of Pranaful. "When you're in the supermarket, focus on the nourishment source," Klein shows. "Hope to check whether it's something that has been created in this country or abroad and endeavors to know about pesticides that may have been exposed to or presented to people who were developing nourishment." If you can, make successive adventures to your neighborhood ranchers advertise, where most sustenance is developed locally, she recommends.

- **Stage 3—Enjoy the preparation process.** When you get ready for sustenance, instead of looking at it as an errand or something you need to hustle through, value the process. You can take a great deal of pleasure in food shopping for items that you know will help you feel better and nourish your body.

• **Stage 4—Simply eat.** This is something we once in a while do, as simple as it sounds, "Simply eat." "Individuals regularly eat while doing different things—taking a gander at their telephones, TVs, PCs, and books, and mingling," claims Dr. Rossy. "While cautious eating can happen when you're doing other stuff, endeavor to' simply eat' at whatever point plausible." She includes that centering the nourishment you're eating without preoccupation can make you mindful of flavors you may never have taken note of. Yum!

• **Stage 5—Down your utensils.** When you are done eating, immediately put your dishes and utensils away. This is a way of signaling to yourself that you are done eating (it tends to be much a bit tough to accept). "You're getting a charge out of each chomp that way, and you're focused on the nibble that is in your mouth right now as opposed to setting up the following one," Klein says.

• **Stage 6—Chew, chew, chew your food.** Biting your sustenance is exceptionally fundamental and not just to avoid stunning. "When we cautiously eat our sustenance, we help the body digest the nourishment more effectively and meet a greater amount of our dietary needs," says Dr. Rossy. Furthermore, no, we won't educate you on how often you've eaten your sustenance. However, Dr. Rossy demonstrates biting until the nourishment is very much separated—which will most likely take more than a couple of quick eats.

Chapter 15 - How to Find the Focus?

How to find the focus needed for gastric band hypnosis rapid weight loss for women?

1.   **Focus on yourself or those things that matter the most to you.** Some people do not usually have a constant partner who will always be by their side during the ups and downs of their weight loss journey. If you are the type that does not have the support of a partner to encourage and motivate you, then this is good, as long as it is not a problem for you. You **can still focus all of your energy on reaching your goals.**

2.   **Focus on your goals and be determined.** This means that you should do your research and understand what it takes to achieve your goal effectively.

3.   **Know what needs to be done first before turning to techniques such as gastric band hypnosis rapid weight loss for women.** You should also set up a reasonable schedule and know how much time you will spend studying or working towards weight loss each day.

4.   Do not quit if you fall behind in your weight loss journey at times.

5.   **Everyone has his or her own challenges in life.** Sometimes you will feel like giving up as you see your weight not going down, but you should also remember to take it one day at a time.

6.   **Find the best support that you can get from friends and family**. Surround yourself with people who believe that you can do it and who are willing to help motivate and encourage you when needed. Take advantage of them by asking for help when needed and accept their good intentions.

7.   Get yourself a job that allows you to work from home if possible so that there will be fewer distractions for you while trying to lose weight.

8.   **Have the right attitude that will help you to reach your goal.** Try not to be too stressed out when it comes to your weight loss journey. You should have a positive attitude that will help you focus and motivate you.

9.   **Eat healthy foods at regular intervals throughout the day so that you do not skip meals and go without eating meals completely.** All of these things will positively affect your progress in losing weight, even if there is a setback or fall off in progress sometimes now and then.

What are some excuses for not losing weight effectively? There are many reasons why people fail to lose weight effectively even with gastric band hypnosis rapid weight loss for women. Some of these include:

•   **Lack of motivation.** It is okay if you do not always feel motivated to lose weight as long as you do not make an excuse to stop doing so. If you think that it is normal for you to be lazy, then this is not a good reason for giving up. You should stay focused and stick with the plan until it is fully achieved.

•   **Excuses about food.** This means that you have the wrong attitude when it comes to food and how much should be eaten at any given time.

You should always be aware of what foods to eat at what times, especially during meals and snacks or when drinking sodas or juice during the day.

• **Depression.** If you are feeling depressed, you should allow yourself some time to work it out. Do not let depression make you give up on your weight loss plans. Try to find a way to escape the depression and move on with your life.

• **Finishing off food or eating leftovers.** You should only do so if there is no other choice, especially during parties or family gatherings. However, you should try to avoid this as much as possible and take leftovers home instead of finishing them off at the dinner table where they were originally served.

Chapter 16 - Portion Control in Hypnosis

A few days before the national holidays begin, there are several who are already preparing to enjoy a weekend of celebrations, a situation that becomes a real challenge for those who have problems controlling their weight.

However, the good news is that, like other uncontrollable desires, appetite can also be controlled through psychological therapies or hypnotherapies with high effectiveness, which would help you enjoy an 18 with no excesses. Hypnosis points out, eating disorders or the inability to control food consumption have various causes. Some factors that could contribute to these eating disorders are low self-esteem, lack of control of life, depression, anxiety, anger, loneliness, and personal psychological factors.

Others are more interpersonal and that can help people to lose control of their diet at an unconscious level, such as family problems, difficulty expressing their feelings and with hypnosis, you can go to the source of the problem, in this case of food. Eat portions on smaller plates and have measures to eat, for example, half of the bread, half of the vegetables, half of the soups, either at home or in a restaurant.

Fad diets usually cause rebounds. Therefore, it is recommended to eat four times a day, and only when you are hungry this can work through hypnosis. Through hypnosis, you can visualize and consume food more slowly. Be clear that in the national holidays the food does not end, advised the professional. Regarding treatment with hypnosis to maintain a nutritional balance, the expert explained that it consists of two stages. First, educate the patient, tell what it is and what the scope of hypnotic therapy is. Second, explain that there is a job on their part.

As for weight control, it has to do with generating the patient a cognitive modification of their brain through hypnosis that allows them to visualize differences in physical and psychological terms and also change the eating habit in terms of the amount of food eaten.

For this, we work with reinforcements, which is where the patient takes audio recorded by the Center for Clinical Hypnosis where there are three levels and thus gradually move towards a new vision regarding what it is and what we eat.

Unlike other methods, the specialist stressed that it does not generate a rebound effect; it is so powerful when people do the work they decide to do what they are taught, such as generating behavioral change, hypnotic work with reinforcement at home, it is a natural way to understand again what food is.

The rebound effect is generated in other instances. With hypnosis, a profound change is generated in the person's behavior and perception of what they really eat for. The important thing is not to mix everything on the same day and avoid canned fruit if you are going to drink alcohol, try it with a light or zero drink, and thus decrease the caloric intake.

How to Stop Overeating

Overeating is a disorder characterized by a compulsive diet that prevents people from losing control and being unable to stop eating. Final episodes last 30 minutes or work intermittently throughout the day.

An excess dining room will eat without stopping or paying attention to what you eat, even if you are already bored. Overeating can make you feel sick, guilty, and out of control. If you want to know how to stop overeating, follow these steps:

Maintaining Mental Strength

Stress managing stress is the most frequent cause of overeating. Regardless of whether you are aware or not, the chance is to make a fuss because you are worried about other aspects of your life, such as work, personal relationships, and the health of loved ones.

The easiest way to reduce compulsive intake is to manage life stress. This is a solution that cannot be achieved with a tip bag that can help with stressful situations.

Activities such as yoga, meditation, long walks, listening to jazz and classical music can be enjoyed comfortably. Do what you must do to feel that you are in control of your life. Try to go to bed at the same time every day and get enough rest. If you are well-rested, you will be better able to cope with stressful situations.

Connect Your Mind and Body Overtime

You can get more out of your feelings by writing a diary that lets you write what you have come up with, talk about your desires, and look back after an overwhelming episode.

Taking a little time, a day to think about your actions and feelings can have a massive impact on how you approach your life. Be honest with yourself.

Write about how you feel about every aspect of life and your relationship with food.

You can surprise yourself too. You can keep a record of the food you eat unless you are obsessed with every little thing you eat. Sometimes you can escape temptation if you know that you must write everything you eat.

Take time to listen to the body and connect the mind and body if you know what your body is telling you, it will be easier for you to understand what will bring you to your anger and manage your diet. Listen to your body throughout the day and give it time to have a better idea about what it needs or wants.

Follow the 10-minute rule before eating a snack. If you have a desire, do not grant yourself immediately. Wait 10 minutes and look back at what is happening. Ask yourself whether you are hungry or craving. If you are hungry, you must eat something before your desire grows.

If you have a strong desire but are tired, you must find a way to deal with that feeling. For example, take a walk or do something else to distract from your desires. Ask yourself whether you are eating just because you are bored. Are you looking in the fridge just because you are looking for something? In that case, find a way to keep yourself active by drinking a glass of water. Please have fun from time to time. If you have the all-purpose desire to eat peanut butter, eat a spoonful of butter with a banana. This will allow you to reach the breakpoint after 5 days and not eat the entire peanut butter jar.

Maintain Healthy Habits

Eat healthy meals three times a day. This is the easiest way to avoid overeating. If you have not eaten for half a day, you will enjoy the fuss. The important thing is to find a way to eat the healthy food you like.

So instead of eating what you want, you feel that you are fulfilling your duty through a dull and tasteless meal. Your meal should be nutritious and delicious.

The method is as follows:

• Always eat in the kitchen or at another designated location. Do not eat even in front of a TV or computer or even when you are on the phone. There is less opportunity to enjoy without concentrating on what you eat. Eat at least 20–25 minutes with each meal.

• This may seem like a long time, but it prevents you from feeling when your body is full. There is a gap between the moment your body is full and the moment you feel full, so if you bite a bit more time, you will be more aware of how much you eat.

• Each meal needs a beginning and an end. Do not bob for 20 minutes while you cook dinner. Also, do not eat snacks while making healthy snacks. You need to eat three types of food, but you should avoid snacking between meals, avoiding healthy options such as fruits, nuts, and vegetables.

• Eat meals and snacks in small dishes using small forks and spoons. Small plates and bowls make you feel as if you are eating more food, and small forks and spoons give you more time to digest the food.

Managing Social Meals

When eating out, it is natural to increase the tendency to release because you feel less controlled than the environment and regular diet options. However, being outside should not be an excuse to enjoy overeating.

You must also find ways to avoid them, even if you are in a social environment or surrounded by delicious food. The method is as follows:

•   Snack before departure. By eating half of the fruit and soup, you can reduce your appetite when surrounded by food. If you are in an area with unlimited snacks, close your hands.

•   Hold a cup or a small plate of vegetables to avoid eating other foods. If you are in a restaurant, check the menu for healthier options. Try not to be influenced by your friends. Also, if you have a big problem with bread consumption, learn to say "Don't add bread" or smoke peppermint candy until you have a meal.

Avoid Temptation

Another way to avoid overeating is to stay away from situations that can lead to committing them. Taking steps to prevent overeating when you leave home has a significant impact on how you handle your cravings. Avoiding temptation means recognizing a high-risk situation and creating a plan to avoid it. This is what you should do:

•   Try to spend more time on social activities that do not eat food. Take a walk or walk with friends or meet friends at a bar that you know is not serving meals. If you are going to a family party that you know will be full of delicious food and desserts, choose a low-calorie or healthy option.

- Try to escape from unhealthy food when you are at a party. Modify the routine as needed. Eliminate or save a little bit of unhealthy food at home. I do not want to remove all unhealthy snacks from home and go to the stores they sell at midnight.

Perform an Exercise Routine That You Like

Exercise not only will make you feel healthier, but it will also improve your mental health and make you feel more in control of your body. The trick to exercise is to do something you like instead of feeling that you are using to compensate for binge eating.

Exercise should feel like fun, not torture. Do not do anything you hate. If you hate running, walking, or hiking, look for a new activity, such as salsa dancing, Pilates, or volleyball. You will have fun doing something you like, and you will get more health in the process. Find a gym or exercise with a friend. Having a friend who works with you will make your training more fun and make you feel more motivated.

Chapter 17 - The Power of Affirmations

"In the same way that rain breaks into a house with a bad roof, desire breaks into the mind that has not been practicing meditation."— Anonymous.

Let's talk affirmations. Affirmations are small little additions that you can put into your life in order to create a life that is filled with joy and is fulfilling. While some might think affirmations aren't useful, when it comes to achieving your goals in life, affirmations are a key that isn't touched upon as much as it should.

But why affirmations? What do they do for you? Read on to find out the power of affirmations, what they are, and why they do so much good for a person, especially when trying to achieve their goals.

Affirmations at the Core

Affirmations are little statements that you say or something that you think. At the core, virtually anything that you say or you think about can be an affirmation. And Affirmations can be both positive and negative.

Do you ever sometimes say things almost involuntarily, or think something on instinct the moment an event happens? Or maybe you tell yourself you'll achieve and do something? All of those are affirmations. They can affect your life in both good and bad ways.

That's the kicker with affirmations. Sometimes you will think something and then it happens. Sometimes you think you can't do something and then boom, like the flip of a switch, you magically can't do it. Or the flip side happens. You say you can do something, and then magically, it happens. Sometimes it's because you tell yourself that you can.

Think of the phrase "I think I can" from the little engine that could. This is an example of an affirmation. Remember that little engine kept saying he could do it, and then lo-and-behold, he achieved his goal! That's because, with the power of positive affirmation, he was able to achieve his goals.

This can create either good or bad experiences in our life because of this. The patterns we use to achieve our goals, the positive thinking that we utilize, all play a focal part in how our lives change, both for the good and for the bad.

Affirmations can be both positive and negative, and if you want to change anything in your life, an affirmation is the first thing that you need to put in place. It is the beginning of a path to change yourself. This is what you're saying to yourself subconsciously in order to help you understand and do something that you will do.

So what are some examples of affirmation? Read below:

- I am responsible.

- I am aware I can change.

- I can be happy.

- I am confident.

322

All of these are examples of affirmations, and this in essence is choosing those words that will help get rid of something and help as well to create something new in life.

The Power of Positivity

When it comes to affirmations, positive ones have a very profound impact on your unconsciousness. Every time you say something you're affirming something. You're affirming that something is this way. So any self-talk, all internal dialogue, and any thoughts are of course a string of affirmations. Affirmations are something you're using at every point in time whether you consciously know this or not. You're affirming any and all experiences with both words and thoughts.

Beliefs that you have been thinking that you've learned when you were younger. For a lot of people, beliefs and affirmations are different. Some beliefs work, but others will limit your ability to create those things that you want. What you want and what you personally believe in when it comes to yourself can be quite different. That's why you need to focus on the thoughts that you do have, and of course, get rid of those that you don't want to have.

You can have affirmations that will benefit you in life. Positive affirmations can magically change your life, but on the flip side, being negative also can have a profound impact on your life. Negative affirmations are something that will change your life, too.

For a lot of people, affirmations can be both good and bad. For example, some people will talk about the issues they have in life complaining about it. Negative affirmations breed negativity. That's why, every time you're angry at something, that's an affirmation that anger will stick around and continue in life. Every time you complain, whine or feel like a victim, that's affirming that you want to be a victim.

Negative affirmations are something a lot of us don't really focus on. It's because we don't think it will hurt us. But sometimes your biggest enemy is yourself, and of course your thoughts. That's because you're affirming the negative feelings that are within you.

Every time you feel victimized, you want to say something about that. If you continue to talk about how you're a victim, you'll continue to feel like a victim. You'll feel like the entire world is against you, and it can be a bit scary and harmful for you. If you feel like your life isn't getting better, look at the complaints you have.

Look at the things you're affirming. If you're affirming that you can't do something if you're affirming that things aren't fair if you're affirming that there are big issues you can't fix, then chances are, you'll continue to breed those feelings.

And that isn't good for you. You need to understand that changing the way you talk and think is the first step, and from there, once you change that, you'll notice things that will change for the better. It's hard to change your thought process, and it can be a struggle. But understand that the sooner you change it, the sooner you use these affirmations for good rather than to complain and be upset, the better you'll be.

This applies to all parts of life. If you want a girlfriend and can't get one, if you keep talking about how you'll never have a girlfriend and you'll never be happy, then guess what? You're not going to be happy! It is really hard to get out of the mindset sure, but affirmations, when you change that, you're not just changing a small thing, you're changing your whole mindset so you can be happier, and have a better outlook on life as a result of this.

Not always One's Fault

You might be reading this and think that it's all your fault for your lot. While to a degree you're the changer of your own destiny and pattern, you probably didn't even realize that your thinking is harmful. Lots of people don't, and you probably never realized how to do this. People throughout different parts of society are learning to recreate their thought processes and create new experiences based on positive energy, rather than negative energy.

You taught yourself to look this way because your parents did, or maybe you were hurt by past experiences, so that's the way you look at these things. It's hard to get out of the trap of thinking this way. But, once you begin to do so, once you start to wake up and realize that your affirmations can be changed, and you'll be able to create your lives in a way that will please you, you'll realize it will help you a whole lot.

It doesn't just work with health and wellness, but we'll go into weight loss and positive affirmations later on, but you can do this with health in general, finances, getting something, your relationships, and love life, whatever you need.

You have to understand that with affirmations; you have to believe in it, and you have to believe it will work. Some people will use these and then think it's stupid, or a waste of time, or whatever it is they want to complain about. But, what will be heard more?

The positive one you've never said, or the negative one that you keep saying to yourself? The negative because you've been saying it for so long. Some say them too few times and then complain when it doesn't go their way, or it doesn't work. If you aren't using affirmations and looking at life with a positive outlook, then you're going to lose as a result of this.

This is a big thing because a lot of people don't realize that affirmations work when you're looking at life positively and you're not complaining and being negative as well. This is a big thing to understand in order to achieve the power of affirmations. They have to be done positively.

And yes, this is a challenge. I totally get that. I know that you probably fall back on the negative, but if you work on trying to be positive, and complain a whole lot less, then you'll start to feel a lot better about yourself too. Saying affirmations is also part of the process. What you do outside of saying the affirmations is just as important. Affirmations work when you're trying to make changes that better your life.

So affirmations are used along with the actions you do. Affirmations are like seeds. You have to plant them in soil that works for them. If you plant them in poor soil that doesn't allow growth that is bred in complaining and whining then guess what? They're not going to work!

If you plant them in the soil where you're fostering growth and wellness, then guess what? You're going to grow it. The more you choose to think about the positive thoughts and affirmations and try to be as positive as possible, the quicker these will work. It is like magic how easy this can be sometimes, so remember this as well.

326

Thinking thoughts that are positive and happy will help here, and affirmations will begin to stick once there is more positivity out there. They are simple, doable, and they can help you really think better about your life and everything in it.

The way you think can change, and affirmations can help build a much better, more positive mindset. But also understand that it isn't easy to put these in sometimes. That's because you're undoing the thought process that you've had for so long, and positive affirmations will work when you give them a positive breeding ground to work in.

The Science behind This

The science behind this is from the realm of psychology because it does work on undoing the thoughts that are there because of prior thinking.

This isn't magic though. You're not going to have a new life magically and the goals that you have achieved just by saying a few affirmations at a time.

Positive affirmations require you to practice and to change the way you think and feel in life. The cool thing about this though, is that it will change you on different levels, and it does have science behind this as well.

Chapter 18 - 100 Positive Affirmations for Weight Loss

George taught Bonnie a hundred useful positive affirmations for weight loss and to keep her motivated. She chose the ones that she wanted to build in her program and used them every day. Bonnie was losing weight very slowly, which bothered her very much. She thought she was going in the wrong direction and was about to give up, but George told her not to worry because it was a completely natural speed. It takes time for the subconscious to collate all the information and start working according to her conscious will.

Besides, her body remembered the fast weight loss, but her subconscious remembered her emotional damage, and now it is trying to prevent it. In reality, after some months of hard work, she started to see the desired results.

She weighed 74 kilos (163 pounds). According to dietitians, the success of dieting is greatly influenced by how people talk about lifestyle changes for others and themselves.

The use of "I should," or "I must" is to avoid whenever possible. Anyone who says, "I shouldn't eat French fries," or "I have to get a bite of chocolate" will feel that they have no control over the events. Instead, if you say "I prefer" to leave the food, you will feel more power and less guilt. The term "dieting" should be avoided. Proper nutrition is a permanent lifestyle change. For example, the correct wording is, "I've changed my eating habits" or "I'm eating healthier."

Diets Are Fattening—Why?

The body needs fat. Our body wants to live, so it stores fat. Removing this amount of fat from the body is not an easy task as the body protects against weight loss. During starvation, our bodies switch to a 'saving flame', burning fewer calories to avoid starving. People who start losing weight are usually optimistic because, during the first week, they may experience a weight loss of 1–3 kg (2–7 pounds), which validates their efforts and suffering. However, the body has very well cheated because it actually does not want to break down fat. Instead, it begins to break down muscle tissue. At the beginning of dieting, our bodies burn sugar and protein, not fat. Burned sugar removes a lot of water out of the body; that's why we experience amazing results on the scale. It should take about seven days for our body to switch to fat burning. Then our body's alarm bell rings. Most diets have a sad end: the reduction of your metabolic rate to a lower level—which means that if you only eat a little more afterward, you regain all the weight you have lost previously.

After dieting, the body will make special efforts to store fat for the next impending famine. What to do to prevent such a situation? We must understand what our soul needs. Those who really desire to have success must first and foremost change their spiritual foundation. It is important to pamper our souls during a period of weight loss. All overweight people tend to rag on themselves for eating forbidden food, "I overate again. My willpower is so weak!" If you have ever tried to lose weight, you know these thoughts very well.

Imagine a person very close to you who has gone through a difficult time while making mistakes from time to time. Are we going to scold or try to help and motivate them? If we really love them, we will instead comfort them and try to convince them to continue. No one tells their best friend that they are weak, ugly, or bad just because they are struggling with their weight. If you wouldn't say it to your friend, don't do so to yourself either! Let us be aware of this: during weight loss, our soul needs peace and support. Realistic thinking is more useful than disaster theory. If you are generally a healthy consumer, eat some goodies sometimes because of their delicious taste and to pamper your soul.

I'll give you a list of a hundred positive affirmations you can use to reinforce your weight loss. I'll divide them into main categories based on the most typical situations for which you would need confirmation. You can repeat all of them whenever you need to, but you can also choose the ones that are more suitable for your circumstances. If you prefer to listen to them during meditation, you can record them with a piece of sweet, relaxing music in the background.

General affirmations to reinforce your well-being:

1. I'm grateful that I woke up today. Thank you for making me happy today.

2. Today is a perfect day. I meet nice and helpful people, whom I treat kindly.

3. Every new day is for me. I love to make myself feel good. Today I just pick good thoughts for myself.

4. Something wonderful is happening to me today.

5. I feel good.

6. I am calm, energetic, and cheerful.

331

7. My organs are healthy.

8. I am satisfied and balanced.

9. I live in peace and understanding with everyone.

10. I listen to others with patience.

11. In every situation, I find the good.

12. I accept and respect myself and my fellow human beings.

13. I trust myself; I trust my inner wisdom.

14. Do you often scold yourself? Then repeat the following affirmations frequently:

15. I forgive myself.

16. I'm good to myself.

17. I motivate myself over and over again.

18. I'm doing my job well.

19. I care about myself.

20. I am doing my best.

21. I am proud of myself for my achievements.

22. I am aware that sometimes I have to pamper my soul.

23. I remember that I did a great job this week.

24. I deserved this small piece of candy.

25. I let go of the feeling of guilt.

26. I release the blame.

27. Everyone is imperfect. I accept that I am too.

If you feel pain when you choose to avoid delicious food, then you need to motivate yourself with affirmations such as:

28. I am motivated and persistent.

29. I control my life and my weight.

30. I'm ready to change my life.

31. Changes make me feel better.

32. I follow my diet with joy and cheerfulness.

33. I am aware of my amazing capacities.

34. I am grateful for my opportunities.

35. Today I'm excited to start a new diet.

36. I always keep in mind my goals.

37. I imagine myself slim and beautiful.

38. Today I am happy to have the opportunity to do what I have long been postponing.

39. I possess the energy and will to go through my diet.

40. I prefer to lose weight instead of wasting time on momentary pleasures.

Here you can find affirmations that help you to change harmful convictions and blockages:

41. I see my progress every day.

42. I listen to my body's messages.

43. I'm taking care of my health.

44. I eat healthy food.

45. I love who I am.

46. I love how life supports me.

47. A good parking space, coffee, conversation. It's all for me today.

48. It feels good to be awake because I can live in peace, health, love.

49. I'm grateful that I woke up. I take a deep breath of peace and tranquility.

50. I love my body. I love that it serves me.

51. I eat by tasting every flavor of the food.

52. I am aware of the benefits of healthy food.

53. I enjoy eating healthy food and being fitter every day.

54. I feel energetic because I eat well.

Many people are struggling with being overweight because they don't move enough. The very root of this issue can be a refusal to do exercises due to negative biases in our minds.

We can overcome these beliefs by repeating the following affirmations: 54. I like moving because it helps my body burn fat.

55. Each time I exercise, I am getting closer to having a beautiful, tight, shapely body.

56. It's a very uplifting feeling of being able to climb up to 100 steps without stopping.

57. It's easier to have an excellent quality of life if I move.

58. I like the feeling of returning to my home tired but happy after a long winter walk.

59. Physical exercises help me to have a longer life.

60. I am proud to have better fitness and agility.

61. I feel happier thanks to the happiness hormone produced by exercise.

62. I feel full thanks to the enzymes that produce a sense of fullness during physical exercises.

63. I am aware even after exercise, my muscles continue to burn fat, and so I lose weight while resting.

64. I feel more energetic after exercises.

65. My goal is to lose weight; therefore, I exercise.

66. I am motivated to exercise every day.

67. I lose weight while I exercise.

Now, I am going to give you a list of generic affirmations that you can build in your program:

68. I'm glad I'm who I am.

69. Today, I read articles and watch movies that make me feel positive about my diet progress.

70. I love it when I'm happy.

71. I take a deep breath and exhale my fears.

72. Today I do not want to prove my truth, but I want to be happy.

73. I am strong and healthy. I'm fine, and I'm getting better.

74. I am happy today because whatever I do, I find joy in it.

75. I pay attention to what I can become.

76. I love myself and am helpful to others.

77. I accept what I cannot change.

78. I am happy that I can eat healthy food.

79. I am happy that I have been changing my life with my new healthy lifestyle.

80. Today I do not compare myself to others.

81. I accept and support who I am and turn to myself with love.

82. Today I can do anything for my improvement.

83. I'm fine. I'm happy about life. I love who I am. I'm strong and confident.

84. I am calm and satisfied.

85. Today is perfect for me to exercise and to be healthy.

86. I have decided to lose weight, and I am strong enough to follow my will.

87. I love myself, so I want to lose weight.

88. I am proud of myself because I follow my diet program.

89. I see how much stronger I am.

90. I know that I can do it.

91. It is not my past, but my present that defines me.

92. I am grateful for my life.

93. I am grateful for my body because it collaborates well with me.

94. Eating healthy foods supports me to get the best nutrients I need to be in the best shape.

95. I eat only healthy foods, and I avoid processed foods.

96. I can achieve my weight loss goals.

97. All cells in my body are fit and healthy, and so am I.

98. I enjoy staying healthy and sustaining my ideal weight.

99. I feel that my body is losing weight right now.

100. I care about my body by exercising every day.

Chapter 19 - Real Life Success Stories of Women Who Used the Power of the Mind to Lose Weight

The first example of a woman who experienced weight loss due to mental power is Dee Chan. She weighed over 400 pounds at the beginning of her weight loss journey. She was in her 50s when she started her journey and had to use curtain fabric to create her own dresses because she could not find any in her size in stores. She also had to wear men's shoes because women's shoes simply could not handle the size and weight of her feet. Chan's weight problem made her feel less than female, a sensation she described as "soul-destroying."

Chan had tried all the traditional diets and weight-loss support groups, but her tendency to overeat, in addition to binge eating of sugar and fat-laden foods like ice cream, kept her from losing excess weight. She even considered gastric bypass surgery but her weight also made that an impossibility as it was unlikely that she would survive the surgery due to her size.

It seemed like all hope was lost until she turned to a clinical hypnotherapist. After hypnosis sessions with the hypnotherapist, Chan was able to change her mindset and thus, stop practicing bad habits like binge eating junk foods. She realized that she was the only one that could bring her weight under control, not participating in the latest fad diet or a gym membership. Her new and improved mindset allowed her to realize that she had the power to control her life and her body. This led to her making several lifestyle changes.

And so, after only three years, Chan was able to lose almost 300 pounds! She no longer had to use curtain fabric to make dresses, nor did she have to wear men's shoes. She could go shopping like the average woman and was able to feel extremely feminine. Because of her success, Chan started training as a hypnotherapist so that she could help other people like herself.

Another example of a woman using the power of hypnosis to think herself thin is Julie Evans. Her husband won an all-expense-paid trip to Hawaii, but the idea did not get Evans excited as it should have. Rather, she got anxious over the fact that she would have to wear a bathing suit. As a stay-at-home mom of 2 with low self-esteem and a sufferer of depression, Evans was the heaviest she had even been at this time, weighing almost 300 pounds.

That trip was a blessing in disguise because it was the wake-up call she needed to get serious about losing the extra weight. She decided to lose weight but rather than go under the knife with gastric bypass surgery; she used the psychology version called the hypnotic gastric band. This allowed Evans to limit the amount of food she ate, crave healthy food options, and lose weight quickly. Within 2 years, Evans shed almost half her body weight and has since then been able to maintain a healthy weight.

These two women are not superhuman, nor did they use techniques that are out of this world. Rather, they started their extraordinary weight loss journeys with a decision to do better when it comes to losing weight and they followed up with mental techniques that have the power to influence their physical health. Any and every woman on this planet has the same capability and power.

A Better Life and Body Starts with a Decision

Living the life you want and having the body you want starts with a decision. Because of being alive, you are going to be faced with many decisions. These decisions have consequences. Being passive and not making a choice also serves as a decision and so, there is a fallout to that as well.

Deciding to join a gym or to follow a particular diet only goes so far if you do not have control over your mind. A decision needs to be made to have complete control over how your body works; therefore, how it sheds weight. The reason that so many women have so much trouble losing weight and maintaining a healthy weight is that they have not mastered control over their minds or mastered techniques that are conducive to maintaining a healthy mental, emotional, and spiritual environment. Good physical health follows the maintenance of these other areas of health.

This is because when we are happier and more fulfilled, we tend to take better care of our bodies. We eat healthier and are more conscious of what we put into our bodies. We tend to take physical activity more seriously, especially when we learn of the euphoric feelings that can be experienced while exercising. There is no going back. Also, when we are unwell mentally, emotionally, and spiritually, the repercussions tend to be felt in our physical bodies and one common consequence is weight gain.

Therefore, the only logical solution to get your body right is to get your mind right first. That starts with a decision backed by your resolve. Techniques for building your mental muscle include:

•   Hypnosis.

- Positive affirmations.

- Using a mantra.

- Using guided meditation.

The benefits of all of these practices have the power to change your life for the better in many ways. The reason the two success stories outlined above achieved these results was because they made a decision that triggered a mindset shift. The processes above are designed to make that mindset shift a positive one that facilitates a weight loss journey. They did not lose hundreds of pounds because of a special diet, weight-loss support group, or special exercise routine.

The reason that these mental techniques helped them and will be able to help you lose weight is that the process starts in your mind. It allows you to have a deep-seated knowledge that you can and will accomplish losing the unwanted weight. With a change in mindset comes the development of new habits and routines that pave the way to success. Hypnosis allowed Dee Chan to change a bad habit of binge eating junk food and adopt a positive habit of eating healthier. That new habit is a large contribution to her success, and it shows that one small change can lead to big results.

Thousands and thousands of women all over the globe from different cultures have benefited from using the techniques listed above to not just become more mentally, emotionally, and spiritually balanced but to take control of their physical health as well. Do not get left behind. You too can experience these benefits. All you have to do is keep an open mind. This book will give you the knowledge and techniques you need. The rest is up to you.

We are not pulling this knowledge out of thin air. The results that can be earned with the power of the mind are not only backed by success stories in modern times, but are also proven by sciences and developed from ancient roots. These techniques did not spring up recently. They have been around for centuries and have been gaining men and women all over the world great benefits, pertaining to weight loss and otherwise, in all that time.

By following the advice outlined in this book with a truly open mind and determination for a better change, you can earn the same kind of massive result that Dee Chan and Julie Evans did. Not only can you lose weight, safely, naturally, painlessly, and sustainably, but you can also gain results in other areas of your life.

Using the mental techniques outlined in this book will be worth nothing if you do not back up that action with conscious and deliberate efforts to make your mind, body, soul, and heart healthier. For example, you cannot expect to eat a pound of cake a day or continue to smoke a pack of cigarettes every day and see the same improvement as someone who makes holistic efforts to improve their whole person.

The same concept applies to your personal and professional life. Many times, women gain weight due to the stresses they encounter in their life. This can be in the form of work, kids, personal affairs, and more. While you may not be about to eliminate the sources of your stress, you can employ techniques that allow you to cope better. Techniques that allow you to better manage stress include:

- Knowing when to say no.

- Taking time out for self-care.

343

- Exercising regularly.

- Eating healthily.

- Engaging in hobbies for pure enjoyment.

I implore you not to wait to practice these techniques, though. Every second of your life is precious and will not be regained after it has been lost. Living life to its fullest potential every day means being healthy enough to do so.

You cannot concentrate as much as you need to at work if you feel drained.

You will not be able to jump, run and hop with your kids the way you want if you are panting because you are winded a few minutes in. You will not be able to enjoy your favorite hobbies and activities without the stamina and energy to do so. Being a healthy weight allows you to have more energy, be positive and be more confident every day.

Start your weight loss journey today! Not tomorrow. Not the next day. Procrastination is your enemy and stops you from enjoying your life and health to the fullest. Turn the page and start your new life in a new and improved body from today.

Chapter 20 - Role of Human Body in Weight Gain/Loss

The human body is a complicated machine, and it gets even more complicated with the many parts that make up the body. Along with all the biological processes that happen in one's body, one will also get hungry. Hunger is often mistaken for other emotions, but its true purpose is to let us know if we need food or not. For example, hunger can be satisfied by eating dinner after having lunch because dinner was skipped in this example. Throughout one's life, we may experience fluctuations of weight related to these urges to eat and their relationship with food intake and feelings about ourselves when we are around food when we are hungry versus being full or satiated.

However, obesity is becoming more of a global epidemic and the weight loss industry is taking advantage of this. Millions of people are looking for a magic diet or a quick fix to lose a lot of weight. It has become increasingly important to understand how the human body works with respect to food and its environment. Understanding how an individual's brain (emotions) is wired and how it interprets hunger can help with weight loss. The human brain is wired to get hungry when it needs food to survive. Hunger is a biological process that has been around for eons, and it is just as important today as it was in our ancestors that lived long ago. Some factors make up an individual and different reasons why people gain weight or struggle with weight loss. There are many diets out there, but one can't forget the type of brain they have when choosing the proper diet for them. Emotional eating or behavioral eating is often a culprit for weight gain.

The human body uses hormones to regulate how we feel, and hunger triggers these hormones to release in response to hunger. Ghrelin is a hormone that stimulates appetite, while leptin is a hormone that reduces hunger. Researchers believe that the reason why leptin and ghrelin levels are low in people who have obesity is due to an impaired sense of satiety or lack of feeling full. This disconnection between body sensations and hunger has become better known as "hedonic hunger." Even though these hormones play an important role in our brain's appetite control, it seems to be one of the main reasons why some people gain weight.

The brain uses sensory cues to tell us whether we need more food or not. Our bodies are always receiving information about nutrition and energy, but this information can only be used by the brain once it has reached a threshold amount. Sensory cues are used when hunger has not reached this threshold, and it is then that the brain will try to make sense of what type of food will satisfy them. For example, if a person is hungry before going to a buffet, they will be more focused on what food they are eating than how much they are eating because their brain needs to know what food will help it fulfill its energy needs.

Since obesity is an issue in our society, dieticians have come up with an estimated number of calories needed on a daily basis for individuals who want to lose weight. However, some people may need more or fewer calories because their bodies are different and can express hunger differently. In order to determine how many calories an individual needs, they must know how much they are currently eating in a day. The easy way of doing this is to write down everything that is eaten for a certain amount of time, like 4 weeks. Then divide the number of calories eaten per day by 4 and that will give you an estimated amount of calories needed to maintain your current weight. For example, if you eat 2200 calories per day, you would need to make sure your new diet plan does not include more than 1800–2200 calories per day in order to lose weight.

There are many diets out there, and people give them all different names. Whether it's called a low-fat, low-calorie, or macrobiotic diet, the basis for all of them is to have a big portion of fruits and vegetables in their meals. In addition to this, most diets are high in fiber, which is important because it helps with digestion. Everyone knows that healthy diets include fruits and vegetables, but not everyone knows why this is so important. Fruits and vegetables are filled with water, which helps quench one's thirst on top of providing necessary nutrients, such as vitamins A, C, & K. The body needs these vitamins to function properly and also aid in recovering from illnesses. Fruits and vegetables contain antioxidants that prevent cell damage caused by the free radicals we get from exposure to pollution or chemicals. It is important to eat a diet that includes fruits and vegetables as well as carbohydrates and lean proteins such as beans, fish, and brown rice. Carbohydrates are an important source of energy for the body because they help the brain function properly.

The human brain is a complex organ, but it needs to be fed in order to stay healthy. Hunger triggers hormones (ghrelin & leptin) to release which the body uses to tell us whether we need food or not. There are many types of diets out there that help people lose weight, but it all comes down to finding one that works for you. Emotional eating and lack of satiety are often culprits of obesity, but understanding why these feelings happen can help prevent it.

Chapter 21 - What Is Self-Hypnosis?

"People mistakenly assume that their thinking is done by their head; it is actually done by the heart, which first dictates the conclusion, then commands the head to provide the reasoning that will defend it."—Anthony de Mello.

Bonnie saw her mother's improvements, and she truly started believing in the effects of hypnosis. However, she was too shy to expose herself to being hypnotized by someone else, even though the practitioner was a professional therapist. For this reason, she decided to practice it by herself. In the beginning, she was afraid of being able to accomplish none of the sessions alone; therefore, she dived into studying everything she needed to know.

After some time, she figured out what the best techniques were to analyze herself, got rid of harmful beliefs, and transformed them into favorable ones. As she was proceeding very well, it is useful to report what information she used to progress.

Self-hypnosis is still considered a mystical phenomenon by many people, even though this technique can be seen as prayer. You are alone and you concentrate on your well-being. If you like, you ask God or a supreme being you believe in helping you. This practice also includes meditation (just like praying does), as well as chanting, mantras, inner confirmation, or affirmation. When you have to perform at work or college, you make such statements like "I don't fear; I'm fine"; "I can do it" or exactly the opposite like "I can't do it. Everybody is better than me," etc. Even when we imagine ourselves in a different scenario from what is currently happening, we are programming ourselves. What you are doing is continuously hypnotizing yourself. Self-hypnosis helps us to come into contact with the unconscious through the use of a specific language, aimed at awakening some parts of ourselves by leveraging archetypal symbols. In fact, unlike our beliefs, words are indeed full of magic, as Sigmund Freud in 1920 says, "Words and magic were, in the beginning, the same thing, and even today words retain much of their magical power." Self-hypnotization is self-programming. Our unconscious understands the symbolic messages of words rather than their rational meaning; that's why figurative language is used in hypnosis for inducing the individual to relax and to focus on the inner world. We are embedding a vivid, information-rich image with emotions in the subconscious mind.

However, we must learn to pray or let's say hypnotize ourselves accurately! Self-hypnosis is the ability to apply techniques and procedures alone to stimulate the unconscious to become our ally and involve it directly in the realization of our goals. By learning the essential elements of communication with the unconscious mind, it is possible to become able to reprogram activities of our unconscious. Self-hypnosis is a method that does not dismiss the support of a professional but has the advantage of being able to be performed independently. This is possible through the use of CDs and DIY courses made by hypnotists to make this practice accessible to a larger number of people with significant advantages, even from an economic point of view!

What Is Self-Hypnosis for?

It was Milton H. Erickson, founder of modern hypnotherapy, who gave an exhaustive illustration of the effects and purposes of hypnosis and self-hypnosis. The scholar stated that this practice aims to communicate with the subconscious of the subjects through the use of metaphors and stories full of symbolic meanings (Tyrrell, 2014).

If incorrectly applied, self-hypnosis can certainly not harm, but it may not be useful in attaining the desired results, with the risk of not feeling motivated to continue a constructive relationship with the unconscious. However, to do it as efficiently as possible, we need to be in a relaxed state of mind. So, accordingly, we start with relaxation to gather the attention inside, while suspending conscious control. Then we insert suggestions and affirmations into the unconscious mind. At the end of the time allocated for the process, a gradual awakening procedure facilitates the return to the state of permanent consciousness. When you are calm, your subconscious is 20–25% more programmable than when you are agitated. Also, it effectively relieves stress (you can repair a lot of information and stimuli you understand), aids regeneration, energies, trigger positive physiological changes, improves concentration, helps you find solutions, and helps you make the right decisions. If the state of conscious trance is reached, if the patient manages to let himself go by concentrating on the words of the hypnotist, progressively forgetting the external stimuli, the physiological parameters undergo considerable variations. The confirmation comes from science, and in fact, it was found that during hypnosis, the left hemisphere, the rational one, decreases its activity in favor of the more creative hemisphere, the right one (Harris, n. d.).

You can do self-hypnosis in faster and more immediate ways, even during the various daily activities after you have experienced what state you need to reach during hypnosis. A better understanding of communication with the unconscious mind highlights how indispensable our collaboration is to slip into the state outside the ordinary consciousness. In other words, we enter an altered state of consciousness because we want it, and every form of hypnosis, even if induced by someone else, is always self-hypnosis.

We wish to access the extraordinary power of unconscious creativity; for this, we understand that it is necessary to put aside for a while the control of the rational mind and let ourselves slip entirely into relaxation and into the magical world of the unconscious where everything is possible.

Immense benefits can be obtained from a relationship that becomes natural and habitual with one's own unconscious. Self-hypnosis favors the emergence of constructive responses from our being, can allow us to know ourselves better, helps us to be more aware of our potential, and more able to express them and use them to foster our success in every field of possible application.

How Do You Do Self-Hypnosis?

There are several self-hypnosis techniques out there; however, they are all based on one concept: focusing on a single idea, object, image, or word. This is the key that opens the door to trance. You can achieve focus in many ways, which is the reason why there are so many techniques that can be applied. After a period of initial learning, those who have learned a method, and have continued to practice it, realize that they can skip certain steps. In this part, we will take a look at the essential self-hypnosis techniques.

The Betty Erickson Method

Here I'll summarize the most practical points of this method of Betty Erickson, wife of Milton Erickson, the most famous hypnotist of 1900.

Choose something you don't like about yourself. Turn it into an image, and then turn this image into a positive one. If you don't like your body shape, take a picture of your body, then turn it into an image of your beautiful self with a body you would like to have. Before inducing self-hypnosis, give yourself a time limit before hypnotizing yourself mentally or better yet, saying aloud the following sentence, "I induce self-hypnosis for X minutes." Your mind will take time like a Swiss watch.

How Do You Practice?

Take three objects around you, preferably small and bright, like a door handle, a light spot on a painting, etc., and fix your attention on each one of them. Take three sounds from your environment, traffic, fridge noise, etc., and fix your attention on each one. Take three sensations you are feeling, the itchy nose, tingling in the leg, the feeling of air passing through the nose, etc.

It's better to use unusual sensations, to which attention is not usually drawn, such as the sensation of the right foot inside the shoe. Don't fix your attention for too long, just enough to make you aware of what you are seeing, feeling, or trying. The mind is quick. Then, in the same way, switch to two objects, two sounds, two sensations. Always be calm while switching to an object, a sound, a sensation. If you have done things correctly, you are in a trance, ready for the next step.

Now let your mind wander, as you did in class when the teacher spoke and you looked out of the window, and you were in another place, in another time, in another space, in a place where you would have liked to be, so completely forget about everything else. Now recall the initial image. Perhaps the mind wanders. From time to time it gets distracted, maybe it goes adrift, but it doesn't matter. As soon as you can, take the initial image, and start working on it. Do not make efforts to try to remind yourself of what it means or what it is. Your mind works according to mental associations; let it work at its best without unnecessarily disturbing it: it knows what it must do.

Manipulate the image, play with it a little. See if it looks brighter, or if it is smaller, or it is more pleasant. If it is a moving image, send it back and forth in slow motion or speed it up. When the initial image always gets worse, replace it instantly with the second image.

Reorientation, also known as awakening, marks the end of self-hypnotic induction. Enjoy your new image, savor it as much as you like, and when you have done this, open your eyes. If you have not given yourself any time limits before entering self-hypnosis, when you are satisfied with the work done, count quietly to yourself from one to ten and wake up, and open your eyes (Traversa, 2018).

The Benson Method

Herbert Benson, in his famous book titled Relaxation Response, describes the methods and results of some tests carried out on a group of meditators dedicated to "transcendental meditation" to reach concentration (1975).

Benson suggested a method of relaxation based on the concentration of the mind on a single idea, which was incorporated in the Eastern disciplines. The technique includes the following steps:

• Meditate on one word, but you can choose an object or something else if you want to.

• Sit down in a quiet place and close your eyes. Relax the muscles and direct attention to the breath.

• Think silently about the object of meditation and continue to do so for 10–20 minutes. If you find that you have lost the object of meditation, gather your focus again on the original object.

• Once the set time is reached, open your eyes stretch yourself well for some additional minutes. Obviously, to perform better, you will need to practice.

Benson proposes this exercise as a meditation practice. In reality, there are no differences between the hypnotic state and that achieved with meditation. This is one of the most straightforward self-hypnosis exercises you can do.

Here is another simple technique that was developed by the first hypnotists because it leads to a satisfactory state of trance in a reasonable time. It can be used to enter self-hypnosis in a short time.

• Begin to open and close your eyes by counting slowly. Open your eyes at the odd numbers, close them at the even numbers. Continue counting very slowly and slowing down the numbering of even numbers.

• After a few numbers, your eyes become tired, and you find it difficult to open them at odd numbers. Continue counting while you can open your eyes at the odd numbers. If you cannot do it, it means you are in a trance.

Chapter 22 - Obstacles to Losing Weight

Being overweight, mainly if you do several pounds to lose as I did, is not just unfortunate; however, it alright could also be perilous. Once I received my top weight of 605 pounds, I used to be informed that I used to be pre-diabetic, which if I were to proceed shortly off, I used to be on, I might not be around for quite a few more years. This fact scared me, and that I realized the time had come to lock in, affect myself, and lose weight so I could affect people around me.

This fact was more challenging than one might expect, in any case, and I realized that this road ahead would not have been just because I had attempted to get healthier before, and I bombed on numerous occasions. I did not know why I had fizzled or how I planned to beat these disappointments to at long last lose the weight and keep it off permanently.

If you do diet previously, odds are this is often a recognizable story. Before I could lose weight, I needed to perceive why I had fizzled yet and what I could do to be fruitful later.

Realizing why individuals come up short with their diets can help you is fruitful by staying far away from these traps. Recognizing what causes individuals to succeed can get you those tons nearer to losing weight and carrying on with a more advantageous lifestyle. To be effective, you understand how to make sensible objectives, fill your diet with entire nourishments, discover an emotionally supportive network, and realize as weight loss isn't a flash. Please find out how to create solid propensities to realize the goal that you can keep it off permanently once you lose the weight and never set it back on.

Weight loss obstruction is one of the foremost widely known well-being grumblings I see. The failure to exercise or diet your weight away is horrendously disheartening. It makes me extremely upset to ascertain individuals full of weight loss exhortation without discovering answers for themselves.

This is meant to be a beginning stage, not a manual. By taking a gander at the most superficial reasons why I see individuals fall through at getting healthier, perhaps you will see yourself, which may help you break the unending pattern of weight loss obstruction.

Obstacles to Losing Weight

You've been trying to lose weight for months, and the pounds just won't come off. It could be that you need to change your diet or workout routine. You may not be sleeping enough or stressed about work. But it could also just be something more complex like a thyroid disorder that is preventing weight loss, which is why it's so important to get a medical examination before giving up on your goals.

Some of the most common reasons women don't lose weight include:

1.   They've already tried a wide variety of diets and are tired of losing or gaining weight on different plans.

2.   They haven't been sleeping well and are stressed about work, family life, and other everyday activities.

3.   They eat too many calories because they lack the willpower to prepare a healthy meal each day at home, go to the gym, or make changes in their eating habits at restaurants and other eating spots out in the world.

4.   They don't like exercising because they are not seeing a payoff for the effort or it's boring and they have trouble getting motivated to work out.

5.   They don't have the guidance, support, or encouragement from loved ones to stay on track and lose weight.

6.   They had thyroid surgery and need to continue taking thyroid medication. Because most weight loss plans recommend sleeping well, eating healthily, and exercising regularly, those who have had surgery on their thyroid may not lose weight like others who think they need to be on the same diet as everyone else in order to lose weight.

Defining Unrealistic Goals

Having a set plan for your weight loss objectives is essential to your success. However, numerous individuals abandon their weight loss objectives because they expect results that need significant investment and determination. If these things were for you before, it could leave you feeling also overpowered to try to do anything by any means. You'll conquer this loss of motion by examination by setting practical, momentary objectives that push your normal ranges of familiarity.

When individuals start to vary how they eat, they set their objectives excessively high and plan to do tons without a moment's delay. For example, I began to get thinner, and I began to construct my solid propensities a little at a time. I gradually cut things like dairy and soft drinks out of my diet against tossing everything out simultaneously.

When you plan to accomplish excessively high objectives, for example, trying to vary your propensities short-term, then possibilities are you'll finish up feeling overpowered and denied. Instead, plan to find how to eating better.

As an example, instead of surrendering beverages totally, discover some beverage options that you simply can without much of a stretch supplant them.

Not Eating Nutritiously

Many people who plan to get thinner commit the error of not eating adjusted healthy suppers. Instead, they either significantly hamper their part estimates rather than changing what they're eating. For some, this suggests eating a diet brimming with prepared nourishments that do not give the reasonable sustenance our bodies need.

When this happens, the body responds, and you'll encounter cerebral pains, fatigue, touchiness, and yearnings. This fact will cause you to either abandon getting healthier or to consume food intermittently voraciously. If you would like to get thinner, you can not merely control zero in on a parcel. You additionally got to make sure that what you're eating is nutritious and your dinners furnish your body with what it needs.

Eating needs to be pleasant, yet when the adoration for food is employed to handle stress in seasons of pressure or misery, it can turn undesirable. If you're an enthusiastic eater, managing the elemental feelings that fuel habitual eating is basic. Care contemplation can assist you with getting mindful of the body's actual needs. Instead of confusing yourself with them, watching your considerations and feelings permits you to interrupt the recurring pattern of passionate eating and choose judicious decisions.

Crash Dieting

Endless individuals find themselves on crash diets to lose weight rapidly. This fact exclusively doesn't work, mainly if you do plenty of weight to lose.

However, it's not economical, so any weight lost on a crash diet will come. Not exclusively does crash dieting not work, yet it can likewise be risky. Individuals who crash diet can see symptoms like wretchedness, surliness, fatigue, and yearnings. Crash dieting can also slow your digestion because you lose muscle, increment your danger of coronary failures if done long-term, debilitate your invulnerability framework, and sustain an undesirable relationship with food.

Moving between various diets or getting thinner rapidly on a careful nutritional plan with no ultimate objective isn't immediate to try to it.

Going on an accident diet will help you get thinner at first; however, the pounds will return after you reach your weight-loss objective. Consider it. If you re-visit the propensities you had before your diet, you'll undoubtedly need revalidation of comparable weight.

Your body needs a constant glucose intake to create your digestion and feed your mind and body with vitality. Crash diets loot your body of this glucose. This fact is often undesirable and risky for you! Ensure that you do sufficient protein in the day, particularly toward the start of the day. Additionally, do whatever it takes not to eat 2 hours before you head to sleep around nighttime. New diets are regular, so dieters get diverted with the gleaming ultimate objectives these diets guarantee to convey.

Diets have claimed that they're going to cause you to lose plenty of weight in a brief timeframe. Individuals will attempt any diet to see whether it works for them. Models are the low-carbohydrate diet, the grapefruit diet, and the cabbage soup diet (beyond any reasonable amount to specify!).

First and foremost, you'll get thinner, yet once the diet timeframe is finished, the weight will return. If it's anything but a lifestyle, it won't stick. Discover one program, which can work for you and stand by it.

Antiquated smart dieting and exercise are the primary way you will find yourself being a drawn-out change that will remain. Learning great bit control is critical. Studies show that individuals who utilize great part control lose more weight than people who don't.

Numerous new diets have pills or shakes that are suggested alongside your great dietary patterns. These are temporarily fixed, and that they cannot be supported for quite a while. Once they are halted, the weight loss will backtrack or end, and almost certainly, the pounds will return.

Absence of Support

Getting thinner and adhering to your diet are often extreme, mainly when there's nobody around you to support you, compliment you on your triumphs, and in particular, be there when challenges gain out of power. Building an emotionally supportive network and encircle yourself with the right individuals are often the difference between progress and disappointment, so be sure you do uphold. Where you discover that assistance is up to you, there's no matter whether it's your family, companions, or maybe online help.

Not Seeing Results Fast Enough

Getting in shape is intense because it can take some investment to ascertain the outcomes. The reason for crash dieting and weight loss pills is so mainstream that they do not work because we'd like to confirm moment results. Weight loss isn't a flash, and it requires significant investment, particularly once you roll in the hay the right way and wish to ascertain enduring weight loss results.

When I lost weight, it required significant investment and persistence. I'll have witnessed a couple of outcomes rapidly due to the progressions I used to be making, yet I even have spent the recent years attempting to get where I am.

Genuine weight loss occurs in steps, and therefore the excursion could be extended, yet as long as you are doing it right, you will not get to move in reverse, and you'll lose the weight permanently.

You Do Not Have Define Objectives

Discover what your objective is. Is it to end at 5k? Is it to lose a group measure of weight? Is it to suit into a dress? As attendants, we generally set SMART objectives. These are objectives that will be dismantled to ascertain whether they are accomplished. It represents:

• Specific.

• Quantifiable.

• Feasible.

• Practical.

• Opportune.

A case of SMART weight-loss objectives is:

• I need to shed 25 pounds before my lyceum get-together on June fourth.

• (This is alright as long because the get-together is more than half a month away!)

Objectives that are not SMART are:

• I need to shed a few pounds before summer.

• I need to be the identical size that I used to be before I had children.

Having these SMART objectives helps you characterize your goals and assess them to see whether you met them. It encourages you to stay zeroed in on what your real goal is. Have a variety and date. Try not to be smug together with your objectives!

Set aside the trouble to line your arrangement for that week. Defining different consistent objectives is often energizing and less exhausting. Multi-week, your purpose is usually to stick to your eating plans and exercise routine, and therefore the following week, alongside the opposite two objectives, you'll move yourself to cycle multiple times. Having things arranged out spares time, and it additionally keeps you from rationalizing.

Diaries are often a fantastic method to make sure that you simply are staying together with your arrangement and maybe an unprecedented way to assess your advancement. There are applications likewise accessible that will help follow along.

Set here and now and end of the day objectives. For your first week, as an example, define the target of removing pop and strolling two evenings after work. Long-haul goals are extraordinary; however, they will be overpowering and baffling. These little objectives are those which will get you to your drawn-out aim in the end. Zero in on them and be available in them. This fact is often an excursion to the improved you!

Don't just zero in on the target of what you would like to lose. Draw your attention likewise to the target of what you would like to select up. Is it a certainty you're inadequate? But, being solid? Have the choice to run a 5K long-distance race? Make sure you truly take a gander at what it's that you got to achieve from your new lifestyle. Making a stable lifestyle and shedding those additional pounds that are terrible for well-being isn't simple. Anybody that comes clean with you, in any case, isn't telling. It takes plenty of assurance and inspiration to stay on track.

By taking the following pointers and applying them to your life, you'll move in the direction of progress and attain your set objectives. Above all, recognize and treat yourself for the difficult work you're advancing to get this going. You'll do it!

Chapter 23 - Weight Stigma

People typically see slim individuals and are dazzled by their self-control, self-assurance, or their determination and restraint.

However, it should be viewed as incredible discretion or extraordinary determination to try not to devour food sources, when you are really not ravenous. It truly is genuine determination or genuine poise when you can try not to eat food sources you don't see at all and you don't receive any prize surge in return.

The plain truth is that anybody would have the option to oppose sweet desserts or any food under these particular conditions, as there is no requirement for any determination or incredible discretion to stay away from food varieties when you are not really eager and when you have no races to stress over. Despite the fact that slender individuals needn't bother with any additional discretion or resolve in these cases, in the event that they do require it, their poise and resolution would work ideally because of the way that they are non-health food nuts.

On top of these limited conditions, calorie counters who need to battle with slimming down of any sort additionally disturb their insight which is particularly viable over their leader work. The leader's work is a cycle that advances and assists with discretion. Thus, individuals who follow severe plans of consuming fewer calories have less discretion and self-discipline in those circumstances when they need more resolution.

Then again, in similar circumstances where weight watchers battle, non-health food nuts have a lot of restraint and resolution despite the fact that they needn't bother with it. What's more, there is additionally another reality. If slim people ate heavenly cakes, sweets, and other attractive food sources, their digestion would consume more calories compared to the digestion state of weight watchers.

The entirety of this implies that slim individuals are erroneously given some acknowledgment for remaining fit and this specific employment comes simpler for them than for those people who keep eating less junk food. These realities lead to the extremely merciless incongruity, which makes it exceptionally difficult to keep getting in shape for people who have been following some plan of consuming fewer calories. Indeed, it is truly conceivable to shed pounds over the long haul, yet a little minority of health food nuts really realize out how to continue to get more fit for quite a long time or years.

Following the pattern, this fight doesn't come without disheartening, stigma, and harms to their attitude that abstaining from excessive food intake does to their physiology both in the short-run and over the long haul. Regardless of the impediments and difficulties, we need to chip away at changing the stigma encompassing weight, particularly weight acquire. You battling with extra pounds don't make you frail in any capacity. The elements that influence weight gain and weight regain have nothing to do with your decisions to eat fewer carbohydrates.

Subsequently, be dazzled by every progression you take, be thankful for each little objective you reach and advise yourself that you are not powerless, yet you are a casualty of an unreasonable fight. This fight is won by a rare sort of people who are more centered on remaining solid than getting thinner, who are resolved to improve their weight not by any fake methods, but rather just in a characteristic way.

The Impact of Weight Stigma

The fundamental inquiry here is whether against heftiness and hostile to overweight mentalities the ones are adding to these results in fat and overweight people.

In the first place, we need to explain this term of weight stigma. It is generalizing or segregation towards people dependent on their weight. Weight stigma is otherwise called weight-based segregation or weight inclination.

One of the significant well-being dangers of weight stigma lies in the way that it can prompt very expanded body disappointment, which is one of the main elements adding to the advancement of different sorts of dietary problems. With regards to the most popular factor prompting the advancement of a dietary issue, it is unquestionably normal and profoundly present romanticizing of being flimsy, as seen in media just as in other socio-social conditions.

In any case, it is never worthy to use any means to victimize someone dependent and weight is one of them. Then again, weight stigma which incorporates accusing, disgracing, and concern savaging people who battle with their weight, happens more usually than we need to concede.

The truth of the matter is it happens all over the place, at home, at school, at work, and at times even in the specialist's office. This reveals to us that weight separation is more pervasive than we think and, as per the most recent investigations on the subject, it even happens more frequently than age or sexual orientation segregation. Another reality is that weight stigma is risky, expanding the danger for various conduct and mental issues, for example, voraciously consuming food, helpless self-perception, and sorrow. Truth is told, weight stigma has been reported as one of the dangers for low confidence, sorrow, and outrageous body disappointment.

Additionally, those people who battle with weight stigma likewise will connect all the more regularly in gorging. They are likewise at a fundamentally expanded danger of building up some sort of dietary problem and they are bound to be analyzed for BED or gorging issues. Those people battling with weight stigma additionally by and large report that their relatives, companions, and their doctors are the most well-known wellsprings of their weight stigma battles.

With regards to relatives and companions, diet talk and weight-based prodding are as a general rule identified with outrageous weight control designs, unfortunate practices, and weight gain just as gorging. This being said, weight stigma in medical services is one more vital concern showing the extent of this issue. The point which shows medical services experts and suppliers, when conversing with overweight and fat patients will give them not important well-being data, will invest insufficient energy with them and will consider them to be irritating, and wayward just as uncooperative with their weight misfortune therapy.

There is likewise an enormous issue in regards to well-known heftiness and overweight avoidance crusades. The consideration is given to weight control and corpulence certainly has soared in the previous quite a while. Thusly, the business has imbued words like eating regimen, stoutness pandemic, and BMI into our normal jargon. Shockingly, since the ascent of these stoutness and weight control crusades, weight stigma has expanded by right around 70%.

These sorts of missions mean great and they are good-natured, by overemphasizing weight control and weight, all in all, they by one way or another support dietary issues giving counterproductive consequences for the general public as a rule.

Weight Stigma in the Media

With regards to weight stigma in the media, during 2017, there was an enormous number of articles distributed in the United Kingdom just as somewhere else that segregate and stigmatize people battling with stoutness or battling with being overweight.

These articles, once distributed, can be drawn nearer by a great many individuals in both on the web and print designs. This is an incredible concern given that weight stigma present in the public eye predicts diverse unfair practices.

Thusly, the significant job of the media becomes an incredible concern. For the foci of the type of segregation, these biased practices profoundly affect both their psychological and actual well-being.

In all actuality, the media depicts being overweight and battling with weight totally incorrectly, which brings significantly more stigma. The media depiction of these conditions which usually is stigmatizing, indeed, it's extremely tricky and persuasive to society's convictions.

Regardless of the worry, editors and distributors once in a while challenge media content by distributing unfavorable articles which fuel weight stigma much more. The significant issue with these sorts of articles is that they

371

generally consider corpulence to be affected by totally controllable way of life decisions which is in opposition to the exact proof which proposes, in any case, expressing that diverse organic, natural, and different variables add to the weight.

These sorts of articles will respect patients battling with heftiness as essentially being too sluggish to even think about getting up and practice expressing that the fundamental justification for them battling, in any case, is their sluggishness.

Articles expressing these things are available by many individuals who begin trusting them whenever they are assaulted by these wrong assertions. Shockingly, when they get out there, they further build up that separation and weight stigma are worthy and they much further support and embrace such convictions. Given that the media have an enormous force and impact on society, it is urgent that their weighty representation becomes a non-stigmatizing temperament.

Lamentably, what we see today is that they don't cling to those moral norms when detailing heftiness. Rather than doing so remembering those moral principles, they consistently advance segregation and weight stigma.

For this to transform, they should be more moral in what they report. When discussing weight, the discussion about genuine individuals and expressing things and guaranteeing their lethargy is the foundation of their battles is garbage with no observational proof to back it up.

Weight Stigma Driving the Obesity "Pandemic"

The following inquiry in regards to this point is whether the common weight stigma is one of those corpulence scourge sources. The appropriate response is yes. In this period of high weight stigma and stoutness commonness, there is certainly a huge connection between that weight stigma culture and corpulence.

For example, there are various examinations led on the subject that recommend that there are various types of weight stigma or weight segregation which significantly more predominant and surprisingly more than separation dependent on nationality and race.

Chapter 24 - Eating

There are various sorts of diets or healthful choices, for example, Paleolithic eating routine, immune system diet, GAPS diet, Okinawa diet, food control as indicated by the investigation of China, Mediterranean eating regimen, irregular fasting, ketogenic diet, detox diet, Montignac diet, diet Dunkan, Atkins diet, macrobiotic eating routine, veggie lover diet, vegetarian diet, etc.

A portion of the weight control plans are upheld by the authority of the academic local area, and others are definitely not. Nonetheless, from my perspective and experience, all are substantially relying upon every individual, second, and situation. Also, we as a whole have a lot to find, including the authority of the academic local area.

All eating regimens or eating guides share something practically speaking, which is to limit food to improve absorption. Also, by improving processing, more supplements are gotten with less exertion. The capacity of our stomach-related framework is streamlined, and well-being is improved. In the world, energy is neither made nor annihilated; it basically changes. What's more, our stomach-related framework changes the energy of food into helpful energy for our body. Burning-through less amount, as long as it permits us to arrive at the energy we need, implies being more manageable with the climate and with our body. Our body turns out to be more proficient in the entirety of its capacities and stays better and more youthful. Furthermore, the equivalent goes for the planet.

However, how would you eat a limited quantity, feel satisfied, be fed, and have energy?

Achievement depends on the ideal blend and preparation of food. That is, adjusted macronutrients and lift micronutrients. The segments of the food and drink we burn through associate with one another. Realizing how to measure and join them effectively, we improve processing and amplify their bioavailability. This will bring us gigantic advantages for our well-being (better nourishment) and the planet (better utilization of assets). A model is as per the following:

Kale, strawberries, corn, eggs, dark garlic, and olive oil Balance the macronutrients of every supper. For instance, as indicated by the sound dish of the model, for a grown-up: 2 bubbled eggs (creature protein has more prominent bioavailability), 200 grams of sweet corn (carbs: starch and sugar), 100 grams of kale (wavy cabbage) rubbed with olive oil (sound fats) and strawberries (nutrients, minerals, and fiber).

Join micronutrients to improve assimilation and upgrade its health benefit. For instance, green verdant vegetables with solid fats. Green verdant vegetables help digest fats, and fats help ingest nutrients from vegetables.

Save work for the digestive tract, eating predigested food. Concerning model: squashed, marinated, kneaded, matured vegetables; yogurt; removed bread; hot proteins; normal sweet food. Recognize physiological and enthusiastic appetite. Furthermore, eat just within the sight of the first.

Take Out Cravings

Envision a situation wherein you could disengage from your longings. Withdraw them and send them away? Some weight decrease mesmerizing frameworks help you with doing this. For example, you might be drawn nearer to envision sending your desires—state on a boat interminably out to the sea. Suggestions can similarly help you reexamine your desires, and sort out some way to manage them more appropriately.

Weight Reduction

The underlying advance of using hypnotizing for weight decrease: Identifying why you're not achieving your goals. How does this function? Routinely, a subconscious expert will ask you requests related to your weight decrease, for instance, requests concerning your eating and exercise propensities.

This data gathering perceives what you may need support working on. You'll, by then, be guided through acknowledgment, a methodology to release up the mind and body, and go into a state of hypnotizing. While in spellbinding, your mind is particularly suggestible. You've shed your fundamental, cognizant character—and the subconscious expert can talk directly to your oblivious considerations.

In entrancing, the trance specialist will outfit you with positive recommendations, demands and may demand that you imagine changes. You can endeavor it right now with our many weight reduction enchanting narratives! Positive proposals for weight reduction hypnotizing may include:

•   **Improving confidence.** The positive proposition will draw in your slants of assurance through enabling language.

- **You are envisioning success.** During spellbinding, you may be drawn nearer to the picture meeting your weight reduction objectives and imagine how it makes you feel.

- **You are reexamining your inner voice.** Spellbinding can help you with controlling an internal voice who "wouldn't care for" to give up heartbreaking sustenance and change it into an accomplice in your weight decrease adventure who's quick with positive suggestions and is continuously adjusted.

- **You are tapping the unconscious.** In the entrancing state, you can begin to recognize the unmindful models that lead to unwanted eating. You can end up being continuously aware of why we are making unwanted sustenance choices and spot control and develop a progressively cautious methodology for making sustenance choices.

- **They are warding off fear.** Mesmerizing proposals can help you with quelling your fear of not gaining weight decrease headway. Dread is a No. 1 reason people may never start, regardless.

- **Recognizing and reframing habit patterns.** Once in entrancing, you can review and examine ways you use eating and "mood killer" these programmed responses. Through repeated positive demands, we can begin to moderate and at last absolutely clear the customized, unaware thought.

- **You are developing new coping mechanisms.** Through spellbinding, you can develop progressively strong ways to deal with the adjustment to the pressure factors, sentiments, and associations. For example, you might be drawn closer to picture a disturbing situation and thereafter imagine yourself responding with a strong nibble.

- **You are rehearsing healthy eating.** During spellbinding, you may be drawn closer to work on making great eating fewer junk food choices, for instance, supporting taking sustenance home at a café. It empowers these steady choices to end up being continuously modified. The training is moreover valuable for controlling desires.

- **You are making better food decisions.** You may need and cherish bothersome sustenance. Entrancing can help you with starting to develop a taste or tendency for more useful decisions, similarly as affect the piece sizes you pick.

- **You are extending unconscious indicators.** Through emphasis, you may have sorted out some way to stifle the signs your body sends when you feel full.

Hypnotherapy urges you to turn out to be progressively aware of these pointers.

Changing Eating Propensities

There are sure ways that we will burn through our food. A portion of these ways are not helpful to us by any stretch of the imagination, and they make more mischief to our bodies. On most occasions, we will, in general, overlook the time factor that eating requires. We scarcely take a gander at the choices that we make regarding food. Everything we do is to decide. Having an eating routine is significant. Nutritionists have instructed us concerning the right approaches to devour our food.

One of them is that it isn't right to drink water following dinner. In the first place, you need to permit the food to settle, and from that point forward, you should just drink water for certain minutes. Then again, they prompt that natural products ought to be devoured before suppers for them to profit your body legitimately. At the point when you devour them along with your dinners, they won't have the effect they would have in the event that you had eaten them before your supper.

The vast majority of these sound realities are straightforward and simple to follow. It's simply that we simply decide not to follow them. Moreover, you will burn through your food sources in those minutes that try not to be burning through it. For example, you will eat a ton of food around evening time, and the solitary action that you will do is to rest.

You will discover that a large part of the food that you eat isn't very much used in the body, and they will, in general, die. The outcome is that you simply wind up putting on more weight because of the helpless eating propensities that you're making.

So reflection will permit you to understand the effect of the choices that you're making concerning food and assist you with changing how you settle on those choices. You will understand that you have some helpless eating propensities and you will choose to transform them for your well-being thus that you will be in the correct shape and weight.

- What are acceptable eating propensities to weight reduction?

- Do you battle to eat well sustenance?

- Do you endeavor to envision you like eating sufficiently, anyway following a few days, you really miss your common sustenance?

- Do you feel that it's difficult to eat well sustenance dependably?

On the off chance that you really need to make keen slimming down affinities, by then, this direct, typical entrancing sound can uphold you.

Additionally, to our "stop solace eating" title, this will change your entire attitude towards sustenance. Unlike the stop solace eating assortment where a huge load of the consideration is moreover on creating mental quality and self-control to go against urges, this assortment genuinely bases on this side of things more—to help you with growing great eating fewer junk food affinities by re-wiring how you think about sustenance on a more significant inner mind level.

You will consider the negatives of eating a disastrous eating schedule. Rather than seeing sweets, modest food, or essentially your favored oily sustenance as charming, you will consider the negatives—the weight you will get, the negative prosperity ideas, and how low and self-fundamental you will feel after you have finished comfort eating.

Chapter 25 - Frequently Asked Questions about Hypnosis

Would I Be Able to Use Hypnosis to Lose Weight?

Weight misfortune hypnosis can assist you with losing overabundance weight in the event that it is essential for a weight-reduction plan that incorporates diet, exercise, and guidance. Hypnosis is generally finished with the assistance of a subliminal specialist utilizing rehashed words and profound pictures.

How Well Does Hypnosis Work for Weight Loss?

For the individuals who need to get thinner, hypnosis might be more compelling than simply eating and working out. The thought is that it can influence the brain to change propensities like indulging. The specialists inferred that hypnosis may advance weight reduction, yet there isn't sufficient exploration to persuade it.

Is Hypnosis Dangerous?

Hypnosis performed by a prepared specialist or clinical expert is viewed as a protected and integral other option. In any case, hypnosis may not be proper for individuals with extreme psychological instability. The results of hypnosis are uncommon, however, may incorporate the accompanying:

Would Hypnosis Be Able to Change Your Personality?

No, hypnosis doesn't actually work by any means. However, that is a pleasant reason. Hypnosis helps with pressure, is beneficial in routines, lack of sleep, quality of sleep, and to the torment of executives, hypnosis can't change character.

How Might I Tell if Someone Is Hypnotized?

The accompanying changes don't generally happen in every single mesmerizing subject, yet most are seen at some point during the daze insight.

- Gaze.

- Student expansion.

- Change in flickering reflection.

- Quick eye development.

- The eyelids ripple.

- Smoothing facial muscles.

- Breathing eases back down.

- Decreased gulping reflex.

How Long Does It Take for Hypnosis to Work?

Contingent upon what the customer's objective is, the customer will show up on normal between 4-12 meetings. Envision for quite a while that you are my customer and that you are sitting in my agreeable "mesmerizing seat."

What Are the Negative Effects of Hypnosis?

There are a few dangers related to hypnosis. The most hazardous is the chance of making mistaken recollections (called confabulations). Other potential results incorporate migraines, tipsiness, and tension. Yet, these normally vanish following the hypnosis meeting.

What Is the Hypnosis Success Rate?

The investigation found that hypnosis had far-reaching changes in six hypnosis meetings, while therapy took multiple times. Furthermore, hypnosis was extremely successful. After 6 meetings, 93% of members had a recuperation pace of just 38% in the analysis bunch.

Does Hypnosis Work When I Sleep?

Hypnosis isn't rest (a contemplation with an objective). However, on the off chance that you are worn out, you can nod off while tuning in to hypnosis. Luckily, hypnosis arrives at the subliminal regardless of whether it nods off.

The Amount of Weight Can I Lose with Hypnosis?

Most examinations show a slight weight reduction, with a normal loss of around 6 pounds (2.7 kilograms) more than a year and a half. Notwithstanding, the nature of a portion of these examinations has been addressed, and it is hard to decide the genuine viability of weight reduction hypnosis.

Does Meditation Lose Weight?

Despite the fact that there isn't a ton of exploration that shows that contemplation can straightforwardly assist you with getting more fit, reflection can assist you with bettering your considerations and activities, including those identified with food. For instance, research surveys have shown that contemplation can assist with both bulimia and a passionate eating routine

Would Everyone Be Able to Be Hypnotized?

In the event that we comprehend hypnosis as an engaged condition of consideration, where there isn't really a deficiency of cognizance or absence of memory about what has occurred in the meeting, the appropriate response is yes. In any case, on the off chance that we comprehend this inquiry as though the entire world can arrive at profound daze (sleepwalking)—comprehended as far as old-style hypnosis—with for all intents and purposes all out suggestibility and loss of awareness, the appropriate response would be a relative NO.

Getting a light or medium daze is generally simple. Arriving in a profound daze is more perplexing; roughly 80% of subjects can arrive at a profound stage absent a lot of trouble. The excess 20% would be troublesome because of a few convoluted factors of knowing or controlling (dread of losing one's inner voice, biases or convictions, absence of trust in the inducer, and so forth) Despite this reality, in the event that we use hypnosis at the clinical level or specialist, as a rule, a medium daze is sufficient to acquire results.

Who Can Entrance?

Hypnosis is basically a strategy. Thusly, any individual who knows it enough and figures out how to apply it can spellbind. Something else is that the inductor would then be able to stand up to and settle the various circumstances that emerge during the meeting.

In certain nations, clinical hypnosis is just permitted to specialists and clinicians earlier approved and arranged.

Would Someone Be Able to Fall Asleep Forever?

It is totally unimaginable for it to occur. Regardless of whether we practice self-hypnosis (about ourselves), or hetero-hypnosis, that is, about someone else, we will consistently wind up leaving the entrancing state. On the off chance that under any condition the trance specialist vanished, the initiated subject would dynamically move from the mesmerizing daze to common rest and would slowly awaken and clear. It happens now and then that the individual is in such a peaceful circumstance that he opposes awakening. All things considered, we can make a counter-idea, for example, "In the event that you need to remain or get back to this state later, you should wake up now"—and will regularly surrender hypnosis. Or then again we just let you rest until you wake up after a period that is normally short.

Does Hypnosis Have Contraindications?

Hypnosis and every comparable state and strategies produce an incredible advantage to the living being since it dispenses with physical or passionate strains, somewhat lessens pulse, controls the heart and respiratory cadence, balances the cerebral sides of the equator and on the off chance that we talk in fiery terms, rebalances the body's bioenergy. Subsequently, on the off chance that we are typically sound individuals, we won't be in any peril. Nonetheless, there are two total signs: by and large, hypnosis ought not to be performed on individuals with schizophrenia or genuine psychological sickness. Why? Since we could bother the side effects separate from each other, which would be hard to initiate. The subsequent case is about individuals with epilepsy or who have had ongoing emergencies of this kind: during hypnosis one of these emergencies could happen, so judiciousness exhorts not to submit them.

Does the Hypnotherapist Have Any Unique Force?

Firmly NO. At the point when hypnosis is utilized as a show, the trance inducer normally gives himself an atmosphere of extraordinary mental forces. This is important for the intriguing climate that the inductor will use to accomplish its breathtaking impacts. Everything relies upon how suggestible and receptive we are.

Truly if an individual doesn't need it, it is hard to be incited, except if there is such a limit dread or conviction that the trance inducer has such (imaginary) power that our own conviction or conviction will make us fall into hypnosis even some of the time immediately to the smallest idea or hint of the inductor. To entrance, you needn't bother with uncommon abilities, yet at least abilities. For instance, a modest, dicey, and uncertain individual would be an awful hypnotherapist or subliminal specialist.

Would Someone Be Able to Be Induced to Do What They Do Not Want?

Albeit a few creators deny this chance, our training just for exploratory purposes shows us that YES. Everything relies upon a wide range of factors, yet in the event that the initiated subject has an adequate level of entrancing profundity, he can acknowledge, in entire or to some degree, the chance of declining the ideas forced by the trance specialist. There have been various cases of assault and mental control under conditions of hypnosis—this is the same old thing. That is the reason we ought not to be entranced by individuals who don't have our certainty.

Would We Be Able to Hypnotize Ourselves?

Obviously. Self-hypnosis is quite possibly the most intriguing part of this strategy. For this, we can utilize—for instance—a tape, where we will record an acceptance to unwind logically, including ideas, for example, "I'm getting more settled, my muscles are delivered, gradually I feel a lovely and profound dream." Eventually, we will add the ideas that we need to execute for different purposes, like concentrating more and better, stopping tobacco, being more settled, and so forth.

Would You Be Able to Hypnotize Us Without Us Noticing?

Hypnosis is more present in our lives than we envision. Truth be told, if this is just a condition of consideration pretty much intense and zeroed in, consistently we endure to a more prominent or lesser degree at least one "hypnosis." Advertising—particularly TV plans to entrance us (propose us) to purchase an item. Government officials utilize exceptionally elaborate correspondence and picture procedures to catch our consideration, even when the last impression is a higher priority than the actual discourse. In any case, getting back to old-style hypnosis, there are subconscious methods to actuate a subject to entrancing states and instigate him/her, without the requirement for loss of awareness—to certain conduct or disposition.

Is There Instant Hypnosis?

Indeed. For instance in mesmerizing shows, when the inductor understands that somebody among his crowd is truly suggestible and even shows some dread when moving toward him, his own dread and the way that the trance inducer is seen wearing an extraordinary force, will make its smallest trace, the watcher quickly falls into hypnosis (ordinarily it will be a light or medium daze and should be extended). The other case would be when whenever acceptance is accomplished, the subject is left embedded with a post-mesmerizing request, for example, "when you awaken and on the following events when I advise you, you will quickly fall into this equivalent state." In the event that the accomplished state is adequately profound, it is embedded in the subject's profound mind and can last in any event, for an inconclusive period.

Chapter 26 - Learn to Fall In Love with Exercise

Welcome to your weight reduction spellbinding meeting. This one is designated "Learn to Fall in Love with Exercise." During this exercise, I will direct you through a reflective excursion and help your body and mind easily comprehend the addictive idea of exercise. Likewise, with most entrancing, you may find yourself shipped into an alternate degree of harmony, a condition of total unwinding. Your mind, body, and consideration will be totally assimilated. Prior to commencing, if it's not too much trouble, ensure you are in a protected, calm climate and not performing any errands that require your consideration like driving or working close to well-being dangers. Preferably, you ought to be giving this entrancing meeting your full, full focus for the most ideal outcomes.

At the point when you are prepared, subside into a decent headspace, and unwind as I control you through a satisfying, remarkable, and profoundly extraordinary experience. You will find yourself in a condition of profound unwinding, stress-alleviation, solace, peacefulness, and inner force. Be set up to have your whole mindset about weight reduction adjusted and your determination dramatically increased. Before long you will find yourself losing weight normally and easily. This is the force of entrancing. Try not to be amazed in the event that you begin to appreciate losing weight and developing better propensities.

OK, how about we begin. Loosen your body and position yourself in the position that most comforts you. You may decide to be in any position, lying down or sitting up. Whatever loosens up you the most and causes you to feel the most settled. When you're done adjusting your positions, begin to see your breathing, and begin to see that it was so natural to get into such a condition of unwinding.

Tenderly shut your eyelids, feeling them getting heavier and heavier. Now take in and inhale out. Slowly shoot out the entirety of your concerns and feel your strain dissolving. Take another full breath in, and as you breathe out, feel your body sinking further into a condition of total unwinding, and quietness. Every breath you take loosens up your body a tiny bit of touch more.

In the event that you don't feel yourself relaxing quickly, don't attempt to propel yourself, instead, let unwinding clear you away normally. The harder you put in the more effort it is, so unwind and permit harmony to come to you.

As you continue to inhale and breathe out, feel the entirety of the strain in your muscles, the snugness. The tensing disappears. Continue to inhale with each breath out carrying ceaselessly somewhat more if the concern somewhat a greater amount of the uneasiness that is clouding your brain. Practice this mindful breathing and acknowledge what it is making you feel. How loose, and how quiet you can't resist the urge to feel. You are totally loose, your mind is quiet, and your body is very quiet, and you find a sense of contentment, safety, and security.

I need you to zero in on my voice. Let it direct you into a more profound and more profound condition of unwinding. Having something to zero in on can truly help bring you into the mesmerizing state that expresses what you are feeling at this moment.

Following my voice. Imagine that you're standing in a corridor, an unfilled foyer with just an entryway on the opposite side. It's an exceptionally huge entryway with ten locks adorning it. You realize that behind this entryway is where you will actually want to unwind. A spot that brings you solace, calmness, and a protected feeling.

As you approach the room, your unwinding uplifts, and you feel your uneasiness melting ceaselessly. You take a full breath knowing that the lone thing separating you from this ideal room is these ten bolts. These ten bolts that overlap you have the way. As you work to open every one of the locks, you find yourself feeling increasingly quieter. The delicate snap as the locks discharge brings you consistently nearer to being inside that serene room.

Presently imagine yourself unlocking every entryway as I check down from ten. Continue to inhale in any way you can to bring the most solace. Ten. Nine. Each snap is so satisfying. Eight. Seven. You're falling further into unwinding and quietness. Six. Five. You are almost of the way there now, you're so close that you can nearly feel the serene environment of the room. Four. Three. Each snap of the lock is so liberating. Two. One.

You push the weighty entryway open to uncover a space that emanates solace. It feels natural. You can't completely explain why; however, you feel as though every choice you make in this room. Every arrangement you plan will succeed. Each expectation and dream that shows in this room will turn into a reality.

Thus, you think, "I will shed pounds and become a better and more joyful adaptation of myself." You stroll over to a space of the room that feels the most agreeable to you. There is a lounge chair waiting for you. It's delicate, you simply need to sink into it and let the pads gobble you up, encasing

393

you in a case of solace. You notice that there is a book close to you when you plunk down and you open the covers to uncover smooth, cream-hued papers. Grasping a decent pen, you begin to make your weight reduction plans, write down your objectives and observe how you will accomplish these objectives. The pen skims preposterous easily, and soon you find out your whole weight reduction venture, each word, and each instance of contact with the paper. You feel like your arrangement is becoming increasingly genuine. It's as though you are sealing your destiny. You are destined to get thinner.

You are destined to arrive at your objectives. You have solid intentions. You are making fearless choices. You are intentionally making a decision, and nothing can shake the certainty inside you. Presently I need you to begin imagining that when you flip the page, you are writing down the entirety of your #1 exercises. The exercises that support your body and make you more grounded, lighter, better, and more joyful...

Imagine how amazing it would feel in the event that you continue to endure until you arrive at your ideal objectives effortlessly. How pleased you would be with yourself for following through. You realize these exercises will lead you to these amazing outcomes. Exercising reliably will instantly hoist your well-being. The exercises that will lead the route to the body you've generally longed for.

Presently, pick the exercise that you love the most. I need you to envision yourself doing it at this moment. As your body moves, imagine yourself getting ever nearer to reaching your objectives. With every breath, each progression, and each ounce of development, you're gradually filling up with good energy considerations, strength, and happiness. Really envision yourself on the occasion, feel the perspiration dripping down your body indicating the difficult work that you've done. Smell the fragrance of achievement coming consistently nearer. Taste the burning craving to endure and buckle down for that drawn-out delight.

You feel so determined. It resembles your general surroundings disappear and your mind is centered distinctly on your prosperity. Your weight reduction and your well-being. It feels easy, as on the off chance that you are in an addictive daze.

Becoming lighter and lighter and consistently nearer to progress. Recollect it as you exercise. Revisit this feeling at whatever point you fail to remember this adaptation of yourself that can't get enough of exercise, the form that is continuously prepared to act quickly. The form that is determined to accomplish their exercise dreams and objectives. You are reaping the advantages of doing these exercises and reaching objectives. You need to do what's useful for you. You need to buckle down for your prosperity and you are making the choices with the total intention that will prompt achieving your weight reduction, and wellness objectives.

Each time you exercise, come back to this second and feel a similar determination. Let it move through you and push you to significance. Let it take control and make exercising easy and profoundly charming. You will feel yourself becoming fulfilled and have a feeling of satisfaction each time you find yourself exercising.

At the point when you're finished writing down these plans a… you peer down at your paper and you understand that you're writing so irately and visualizing that exercise situation that you've nearly failed to remember you are writing altogether. So easily. You've composed page upon page, ingraining these realities into your brain. Just like how you would feel after an intense exercise meeting. You would think back and be glad and have a positive outlook on what you've achieved. That amazing feeling of satisfaction and fulfillment, you hunger for that and you need that.

You gradually shut that diary, loaded up with your arrangements, and spot it back on the love seat. You'll have the option of finding it here at whatever point you need to audit your arrangements, update them, or be reminded of your objectives. You stand up and advance back towards the entryway. When you leave this time, you leave the locks opened. You understand that the entirety of this determination and strength was inside of you from the beginning. You simply required a push the correct way to open those locks. Now you will be allowed to return to this room. Revisit your diary, revisit these freshly discovered feelings, and love for exercise at whatever point you need to.

I will currently tally down from ten. When I reach "one" you will advise your psyche mind to show these certainties. You will do whatever you need to in request to arrive at your weight reduction objectives. You are in outright control.

Also, nothing will stop you. Ten. Nine. You can hardly wait to begin exercising. Eight. Seven. You can hardly wait to feel that feeling of satisfaction and fulfillment. Six. Five. You can nearly taste achievement and you can assuredly see yourself achieving it through exercise. Four. Three. Two. You're in charge and you are choosing to permit the exercise to get easy. One.

Chapter 27 - Hypnosis and the Metabolic Circuitry for Weight Loss

Hypnosis Clears the Metabolic Circuitry for Weight Loss Counteraction

On the off chance that you are corpulent, you might be worn out on reminding every individual that diminishing weight burns through less food and assimilates fewer calories. Each diet you may have attempted, old and new. Frequently our bodies appear to have discovered a method of transforming a lettuce plate directly into pound additional pound fat!

At some point or another, numerous individuals who need to get thinner discover their efforts confounded by high-impact frameworks that hold weight on the body paying little mind to exactly how one changes its dietary patterns.

In the event that you are hefty, or your dear companion or client, and think about losing some weight, if it's not too much trouble, take the accompanying arrangement of inquiries:

• Can you detect that regardless of the amount you starve yourself, the weight simply isn't decreasing as quickly as it ought to be?

• Do you find that you eat less food than your thin old buddies and still don't decrease weight?

- Will you find that your food desires are additionally going up as the additional pounds tumble off? As though you starved to death rather than on a tight eating routine program?

- Do you wind up idle and tired with regards to food abstinence programs?

- Can you, at a remarkable speed, get back all the weight that you lost from an eating regimen?

Whenever replied "yes" to these inquiries, you likely have some subliminal metabolic programming to clutch your body weight instead of consuming it for power as it ought to.

The uplifting news presently lies underneath! There are various ways that we can handle this hypnosis programming, so you don't have to battle your body to drop weight notwithstanding your longings for food!

At first, the reasons for this programming will be taken a gander probably, conceivably. Food digestion is a complete instrument by which the body retains supplements from food and utilizes them. It is a perplexing interaction, including a few variables.

One is the capacity of the thyroid gland, the "ace catch," which through mesmerizing symbolism, controls the pace of the metabolic interaction we can show thyroxin advancement, the essential metabolic chemical delivered by the thyroid gland.

More thyroxin makes the fat be liquefied, prompting weight loss and more energy for you. There might be clinical clarifications for a thyroid condition, which is the reason we suggest an exhaustive actual assessment and plausible screening of your thyroid capacity before hypnosis preparation.

The action of 2 fundamental pancreatic chemicals is an extra key factor in the metabolic cycles of the body: insulin and glucagon. These essential metabolic, hormonal specialists cause us to store or shed fat in our bodies. The kinds of food you eat can impact certain hormonal specialists' exercises. In an essential, most carbs, including sugars, will instigate insulin discharge, which builds sugar digestion and capacity.

Glucagons, which are delivered after a diminished carb dinner, help multiprotein and fat in the body. This is important for why low carb eats less come to be liked.

How does hypnotherapy help transform your food decisions? Since all food ceremonies are inserted in the psyche mind, regularly deciding to eat in different ways is sufficient to make long-haul customizations in our dietary patterns. The hypnotherapy picture addresses and changes these subconscious cycles in a manner that is both perpetual and almost effortless. For a reality, adapting to mental eating designs is of crucial significance. Scientists have found routine exercise, as low as 30 minutes per day.

Mesmerizing thoughts can be utilized to improve one's inspiration to rehearse just as to upgrade force and endurance. However, frequently, it takes considerably more than straight entrancing plans to get more included again with the exercise.

One of the astute cycles that we use is to return you to what you in a real sense appreciated doing as a youngster. You can pick a couple of those exercises which you will certainly appreciate indeed! We utilize the force of hypnosis to restore the perky satisfaction you encountered as a child. We can return to those horrendous encounters that set off us to kill to practice bliss and free the previous self from these wounds.

For instance, a piece of information about being denied, embarrassed, or hurt in the jungle gym in a group activity can prompt one to close down the need to play outside. Our salvage target permits the youngster to acquire comfort from the adult self and a guarantee of well-being and security, alongside a challenge to play outside with an experienced childhood in another climate.

One of metabolic programming's shared devices is innate. Some human hereditary lines (South Pacific Islander and Eskimos offer just two limit models) keep fat on their bodies quicker on the grounds that these highlights conveyed well to their forefathers, particularly in the midst of starvation. It very well might be hard for equipped experts to change those hereditary codes inside our DNA.

Through Hypnosis, in any case, we can persuade the metabolic rate to sidestep certain DNA projects and help us discharge fat. My customers have regularly said to me, "My whole family is corpulent!" This is an ideal opportunity to utilize subtleties of entrancing suggestions pointed toward bypassing DNA shows.

Another regular subject for those who manage weight loss is that the psyche brain can be terrified. Given that if one of the weight loss problems goes away, the weight loss may need to experience other ways to make all the problems scarcer.

Another lady, in hypnosis, revealed to me that in the event that she lost the weight she acquired, she would need to "take care of my life, and I don't understand what to do!" At the Institute, we will check for these issues and have a treatment plan. One valuable methodology that can be utilized from underneath is a way into the future self to sort out some way to satisfy one's life effectively.

Another regular thought process that I have found among ladies customers with metabolic shows to store fat is the need of the body to protect itself from undesirable sexual improvements by utilizing fat. The vast majority of my corpulent customers are casualties of lewd behavior by young fellows.

A few others have put on weight inside an unfulfilled union due to their neglected sex-related demands. Many blame weight for not gathering men, and therefore risk being dismissed or beguiling. At the point when you are new to these subliminal frameworks, you can be covered somewhere down in the psyche's mind and might be influencing your digestion. Your hypnotherapist will assist you with finding the issues and reestablish them. I was by and by powerful in saving customers from early rape injury, which regularly brought about emotional weight loss with no noticeable dietary improvement.

Quick Weight Loss and Fast Diet

Great and Bad Hypnosis

Hypnosis is superb, terrible, and not terrible, but not great either. Indeed, even in this day and age of hypnosis, there is a great deal of poop out. I do accept that there is some astounding roundabout worth of hypnosis (particularly situations); my sincere belief is that circuitous/conversational hypnosis is, by a wide margin, on the "razor's edge" as it is currently, as proficiency and exceptional.

Be cognizant on the grounds that various hypnosis shills sell objects of mesmerizing scams, for example, low-rate subconscious prompts and stuff of pseudo-otherworldliness. Try not to misunderstand me, I'm not against every one of the subconscious cues, and I figure hypnosis ought to be utilized when joined with otherworldliness.

It Is Feasible to Entrance Even Passionate Quitters/I Cannot Be Hypnotized

You may have heard that you can't entrance "shrewd" individuals. Numerous individuals don't believe that sort of stuff to be fun, and so they simply don't get into hypnosis. It is principal.

Then again, in the event that you experience being marvelously and delicately guided into a condition of profound unwinding and fixation, you can understand that you can be spellbound. It's feasible to spellbind somebody with sound mental teachers and a reasonable measure of knowledge.

Truth is told experience shows that individuals who are sharp and have an innovative psyche make the absolute best subjects/customers for hypnosis since they can "accept past the container" and don't limit their minds to what exactly is feasible for them.

Hypnosis Is the Force of Grade/You Are Not the Captive of the Subliminal Specialist

You are the one in particular who has full control over your psyche. A therapist can't allow you to do whatever you will not do. This fantasy has been spread for excessively long by bizarre paper reports, stage hypnotherapists, and individuals who don't understand much about hypnosis.

This being said, an individual may utilize procedures of hypnosis and influence (for both amazing and unfavorable capacities) to make another individual end up bound to do what they say and to follow their ideas.

Everybody can settle on their own choices (considerably under hypnosis) at last; however. A trance inducer can't request that somebody do anything without wanting to (counting conflicting with his/her ethics) except if he/she is really able to do as such from the outset.

When all is said in done, the therapist fills in as a manual for bring you into a quiet and focused state and uses intellectually solid entrancing strategies to help you make changes or experience various things you need to encounter.

Hypnosis Is Not Resting

Despite this theory, individuals who first attempt hypnosis now and again emerge from it somewhat frustrated. They make statements like, "I could hear whatever you said" or "I felt like I could open my eyes and leave if I needed to." indeed, in the event that you stay in hypnosis, you will be aware of your environmental factors. The expression "Rest!" is typically utilized by trance specialists as a request to force somebody into a daze. It is the way it utilizes rest as an instrument to assist us with getting hypnosis.

In Hypnosis, You Cannot Get "Stuck"

Nobody got trapped in hypnosis. The solitary explanation an individual ought to stay in a daze is that it feels beautiful to be so loose and thought. In the event that the trance inducer left or abruptly passed on while the individual was in hypnosis, the most noticeably awful thing that would happen is that the mesmerized individual would presumably drop off to rest and stir a truly extraordinary inclination.

Chapter 28 - Weight Loss Journey

The weight loss journey is certifiably not a simple way to take. It's an enormously daunting task that begins with the brain. You need to figure out how to be sure about yourself and your body to have a solid change. Fortunately, spellbinding is here.

Spellbinding is a fantastic method of mending the psyche since when you're centered around something different, you can't harp on the entirety of your negative contemplations and stresses that are demolishing your everyday life. So it's a fantastic method to begin your new weight loss routine.

The best ideal opportunity to begin the entrancing is in the first part of the day since you will be engaged and can become familiar with your new propensities effortlessly. To start, track down a tranquil spot where you can unwind and zero in on yourself. Ensure nobody interferes with your meeting or occupies you since this may demolish the entire interaction. When you're prepared, the journey can start. You'll feel great and arranged to become more acquainted with your new body.

You may feel somewhat peculiar from the outset, yet you'll just be in this state for several minutes, so it's a sorry issue. You can likewise go with entrancing before bed and wake up feeling invigorated and prepared to begin the day.

• **Stage 1:** The enlistment stage is the point at which you will be guided into spellbinding with strategies. For example, representation works out, guided symbolism, and self-entrancing.

- **Stage 2:** The subsequent stage is the point at which your psyche brain will be offered guidelines to dispense with every one of the negative sentiments in regards to your body.

- **Stage 3:** The last stage is the point at which you will be guided into a condition of profound unwinding with the goal that your body can eliminate all contrary energy and acknowledge another, better character.

To get in shape through spellbinding, you should give it all that you have and take the necessary steps to get results, regardless of whether it implies following an exacting eating routine made, particularly for you by your primary care physician. This will guarantee results and not simply weight loss; remaining fit. I promise you will finish this cycle since it will be simple, and you'll have another body that accommodates your way of life now. It's the most effortless approach to dispose of negative routines and start another you.

The interaction is clear since it is an abstract technique and can be utilized by anybody. You simply need to follow these means. Keep in mind, "you needn't bother with outrageous weight loss entrancing for ladies; you simply need a little assistance."

My Weight Loss Journey—How I Lost 100 Pounds

"Today, I'm 100 pounds lighter than I was where I started my weight decrease adventure." My story isn't one of the overnight accomplishments. I didn't take a magic pill.

My results were not from a rage diet or a thing from an infomercial. My outing has been more like an insane ride of starters, various mix-ups, and a combination of little accomplishments in transit, in the end provoking more than I anytime expected to obtain.

I was a dismal young woman with no certainty, gotten under a free shirt and stretchy jeans and critical to persuade fit as a fiddle to be run of the mill just. I did not understand that it would change into an outing of self-exposure, opportunity, and finding delight. Thoughtful no uncertainty, and 100-pound weight decrease.

Diets I Tried on My Weight Loss Journey

Over the various significant lengths of endeavoring to get more slender, I attempted different weight-loss diets, programs, and shockingly a couple of stunts.

I wish I had been adding to a blog while I'd been on all of them. Nonetheless, I endeavored many of them when I was young, so there is no put-down record of my experience. Here are only a couple of the numerous things I attempted:

- Slim-fast.

- Atkins.

- Squeezing.

- The whole 30.

- Weight loss pills.

- Weight watchers.

- Abdominal muscle belts.

- Stomach contracting wraps.

- Calorie tallying.

- Skipping suppers.

Growing Up As the Fat Kid

I was a charming child until first grade. I don't have even the remotest clue why I started glutting, regardless. I was conceivable on the grounds that I was a daddy's youngster, and I expected to remain mindful of his pieces to be actually similar to him.

Possibly, I was willful and understood my mother expected to eat overwhelmingly, so I revolted by sneaking awful sustenance. Possibly I appreciated food (and still do!). On the day after I was considered, my mom communicated, "It seems like you just need to eat ALL the time!"

Whatever the clarification, I started pigging out and just couldn't stop. I recall my grandmother saying something once about how dazed she was that I could eat incalculable such cuts of pizza. Also, I felt satisfied with having the choice to do accordingly.

I venerated crummy sustenance and would sneak into the kitchen late around evening time and find the unhealthiest food my mom had stowing away in the kitchen, and I'd eat everything at a time. Whether it was an instance of Nutty Bars, a sack of chips, or some really tasty additional items, I'd gobble them up.

Food (even more expressly, poor sustenance) was a significant thing to me. At the point when it was there, I slanted that it was a resource that could run out at some arbitrary time, so I expected to eat everything as fast as possible before someone else set off to endeavor it themselves and leave less for me. I was essentially like Joey from Friends. "Becky doesn't share food!" Aversion I was anytime denied.

My mother was (and still is) a remarkable cook. She for the most part made a tremendous heap of delicious, sound, locally developed dinners; in any case, I never esteemed them. I was constantly requesting arranged food assortments, prepackaged food sources, and modest food.

I would have taken a lunch over a sandwich rapidly and wished I could live off doughnuts, potato babies, and cupcakes. I strikingly review wishing someone would replace all water fountains with Kool-Aid wellsprings (fun fact—I didn't start adoring plain water until I was 27 years old).

The Opposite Extreme

That year, I turned out to be pitifully enchanted. We dated, we prepared for marriage, and subsequently, he was sent, and I lived in a consistent state of pressing factor. I drifted to the following ridiculous of bothersome weight decrease. I was miserable. I thought focusing was the single thing I could offer at that point, and since I couldn't handle what was occurring abroad, I decided to control my eating. I was living alone and, for the vast majority of that year, I apparently ate between 500–800 calories consistently.

I was voracious, an incredible arrangement, not rehearsing using all means, had no energy, and my stomach was persistently in tangles. At this point I shed 40 pounds, bringing me down to 160. That was the lightest I'd been since I could review (from a flat-out perspective. I expected to have been 160 pounds eventually in my life as I was gaining the weight. Nonetheless, I have no idea about when that was). I thought slim suggested sound, yet despite the fact that I was, finally, a common weight, I was far from strong by that point.

Grievous Relationship—Unhealthy Body

The course of action was completed. He got back, and we got hitched. I was ready for a charming specific first-night stage. In any case, it was definitely not a happy or decent marriage.

I didn't have any colleagues with it by then. However, my significant dangers from being the fat youngster mixed in with that earnestness for thought from people had driven me into a genuinely harsh marriage. My weight decrease as adventure spiraled down, and my weight shot up to be sure.

We are a huge burden of modest food, occasionally glued to our TV and PC screens, and the pressure factor of constant conflict between us was practically horrendous for this human fulfilling, agreement venerating young woman!), so I started recuperating the weight quickly.

As of January 2012, I weighed 194 pounds. I started buying more humble articles of clothing and seeing that things fit me such a ton better, yet it was brief. I'll exercise in secret. Thusly, I joined a rec focus.

I was really only content with using the bent. I was too terrified to even consider evening consider endeavoring any of the classes offered, and the weight machines were essentially frightening. Rec focus people reliably seem to comprehend what they're doing and I just... didn't.

I didn't feel like I fit wherever. I especially didn't require people to see my activity place inadequacy, so I put a huge load of energy in the cardio film room, where the sum of the lights is decreased. They projected movies onto a screen before the cardio gear. I endeavored a wellness mentor for a spell and despised it.

The individual who watched me practice was the most horrendous. Mostly because of the weight light. I began working out with a weight she gave me; she reliably conveyed to me how stunned I was at how little I could lift/push/squat/whatever. Despite the fact that I weighed 55 pounds, which was unequivocally not my heaviest weight, I felt inadequate and waited for it to slip away.

That is when I decided to start running. Surely, running. My weight loss journey has been such a great deal greater than 100 pounds. It gave me the opportunity and such profound bliss. I figured out how to exchange my blame for God's beauty. It improved my connections. I feel such a ton better. It supported my certainty. I figured out how to discover happiness and fulfillment in restraint. I improved my relationship with God and others. It transformed me into one that I am frantically infatuated with living.

Also, presently, I need to offer that to others. I need you to understand that, paying little heed to what your starting spot is, you can find that chance as well.

Conclusion

Thank you for making it to the end. Rapid weight loss, or "weight loss hypnosis," is a new concept that has many wondering if it's just another fad diet. Many weight-loss programs involve learning the importance of controlling your emotions in order to create long-term success.

Emotional eating can result in weight gain at any time, so understanding how to manage feelings and improve personal relationships should be a cornerstone of any successful plan. Naturally, when something is unique and different from what has been done in the past, people have concerns over its effectiveness. Weight loss hypnosis addresses this concern by helping people become aware of the power they have over their own emotions.

Weight Loss Hypnosis is a popular weight-loss tool that is used in many variations across the board. From self-hypnosis tapes to weight loss hypnotherapy, this system has been proven to be effective in helping people achieve their goals. Most people are using it in conjunction with other methods that are designed to create balance and harmony within the mind—including meditation, affirmations, visualization, and a healthy diet.

Weight Loss Hypnosis is based on a simple realization: If you can change your thoughts, you can change your life. The use of hypnosis as a tool has been proven to work over and over again. This is why Weight Loss Hypnosis uses hypnotherapy (a controlled state of being) to help you overcome emotional eating patterns and develop positive beliefs about food.

There are several ways that people use hypnosis to lose weight:

• Hypnotic or therapeutic hypnosis is a form of self-hypnosis that involves the use of the hypnotist for guidance, assistance, suggestions, and support. It is most often used by professional psychologists, psychiatrists, physical therapists, and other health professionals who are trained to do so. Hypnotic or therapeutic hypnosis rarely, if ever, is used to lose weight.

Hypnotist

A hypnotist is a person who induces a state of hypnosis by means of various techniques. The hypnotist can be a professional or simply someone who has mastered the art of inducing hypnosis in others. Sometimes this person may also be a psychologist, physician, physiotherapist, or other health professional trained in clinical hypnosis. Hypnotists are often hired by such professionals to help their patients learn self-hypnosis as well as for use in group meetings and seminars. This form of hypnosis is not used to lose weight but it can help people quit smoking and many other self-esteem issues.

Hypnosis is the use of a subconscious mind state to facilitate healing. This is also known as guided imagery and it's used by many people for a variety of purposes, including weight loss in some cases.

Self-hypnosis, as the name implies, uses hypnosis to help you go into a hypnotic state yourself. Because you are in control, this form of hypnosis requires more effort on your part but with proper use, it has proven itself to be very effective. This can be done through television broadcast via home video or audiotapes or even by using an MP3 player with earphones so that you can listen to your self-hypnosis in privacy.

The reason why Weight Loss Hypnosis works is that it allows you to remove your conscious mind from the decision of consuming food. This means that regardless of whether you are hungry or not, you will still have a craving for the food. In doing so, it achieves the same result as hypnotherapy—allowing you to reprogram your subconscious mind so that it releases control over eating habits and gives back the power to your conscious mind. The best way to deal with emotional eating or weight gain is to stop relying on willpower alone and instead learn how to manage negative feelings that lead to overeating.

Many people are under the impression that hypnosis is like sleeping or unconsciousness. However, successful weight loss hypnosis will never put you to sleep; it puts you in a relaxed and focused state of mind, where your subconscious believes everything you say. This can help you lose weight and release toxins from your body by changing your negative eating habits and thoughts towards food.

The use of hypnosis for weight loss may be the best way to address emotional eating because it allows you to be aware of what's going on emotionally while working on your conscious decision-making process. By having a distraction-free environment, you can be in control of your mind and body so that you will be able to stop emotional eating without giving it power.

Self-hypnosis has a proven track record of helping people lose weight as well. So why would you choose to try weight loss hypnosis instead? The reason is simple: With weight loss hypnosis, there are no general guidelines or rules on how much weight you should lose or how often you should work out. From the moment hypnosis begins until it's completed (usually 60 minutes), things like stress and emotions are kept under control. You won't have any instructions designed to make people feel guilty for eating or forcing them to exercise for an extended period of time. Instead, you work on your own willpower to make changes. If you're serious about making a lifestyle change, Weight Loss Hypnosis can help you each step of the way.

417

Lightning Source UK Ltd.
Milton Keynes UK
UKHW020711141222
413914UK00014B/809